Slow Dance

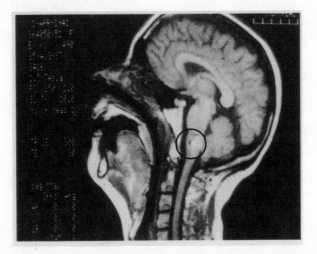

MRI reveals a circumscribed, solitary, intra-axial, vascular, expansive lesion—typical of a cavernous angioma. The pt's neurological condition and the location of the lesion would make a direct, open operation extremely hazardous.

Slow Dance

A Story of Stroke, Love, and Disability

BONNIE SHERR KLEIN

in collaboration with
Persimmon Blackbridge

PAGEMILL PRESS
A Division of Circulus Publishing Group, Inc.
Berkeley, California

Slow Dance: A Story of Stroke, Love, and Disability
Copyright © 1997, 1998 by Bonnie Sherr Klein
Originally published by Alfred A. Knopf Canada, a division of
Random House of Canada Limited, Toronto, Canada.

PUBLISHER: Tamara C. Traeder
EDITORIAL DIRECTOR: Roy M. Carlisle
COVER DESIGN: Big Fish Design
INTERIOR DESIGN: Circulus Publishing Group, Inc.
TYPESETTING: Holly A. Taines
TYPOGRAPHIC SPECIFICATIONS: Body text is set in 11.5/16 Sabon;
journals in 10.5/17 Novarese; additional voices in 12.5/15 Perpetua;
and medical notes in 11/16 Gill Sans Light. Novarese and EvaAntiqua
Light are used for display.

Printed in the United States of America
Library of Congress Cataloging-in-Publication Data
Klein, Bonnie Sherr.
    Slow dance : a story of stroke, love, and disability / Bonnie Sherr
Klein ; in collaboration with Persimmon Blackbridge.
    p.   cm.
ISBN 1-879290-15-4 (hardcover : alk. paper)
1. Klein, Bonnie Sherr—Health. 2. Cerebrovascular disease—Patients—
Canada—Biography. I. Blackbridge, Persimmon, 1951- . II. Title.
RC388.5.K584   1998
362.1'9831—dc21 [b]   98-29017 CIP

The quotation on page 249 is from *Ton Numéro,* a poem by Gérald
Godin in his *Ils ne demandaient qu'à brûler.* Copyright © 1987,
L'Hexagon. Translated by Bonnie Sherr Klein.

Distributed to the trade by Publishers Group West
10 9 8 7 6 5 4 3 2 1

For Michael,

and for all the family and friends
who pulled us through.

❋ Contents ❋

❋ Preface ❋

Ten years ago, if I were setting out to make a film about catastrophic illness and subsequent disability, I would not have cast myself in the lead role. In my pre-stroke ignorance, I probably would have looked for someone stronger and braver than I—not yet knowing that we are all capable of much more bravery than we think.

I would have written a "heroine" who did not have the financial advantages that I have. She would have been younger—in her twenties or thirties—which is more typical with congenital strokes like mine, before she had had a chance to build a life and family of her own. I certainly would not have chosen that she be married to a physician, as I am, who could challenge and when necessary manipulate the medical system to take care of his wife. People might rightly say: What would have happened if her husband had not been a doctor, had not known what and whom to ask? We can't deny the access and resources we had as a medical family. On the other hand, through our story people can see that medicine, even when well-meaning, is not infallible or always humane or even wise.

But Life gets in the way of Art; the role was cast upon me, and I've played it the best I can.

Surviving the stroke has been the most challenging and creative project of my life. There were no guides or maps. I had never known anybody as sick as I was. For the first three years I was isolated with no role models. It was both scary and exhilarating. I was inventing every moment, as in the best of documentaries, with no script.

After my first, relatively mild, stroke, and even after the devastating second stroke that totally transformed my life, friends would say, "Someday, when all this is over, you will make a film or write a book about it." This message, meant to be reassuring, instead made me upset and angry. Somehow, their words seemed to trivialize what I was living. My life is not just raw material for my work—or is it?

Despite my resistance to that idea, I did start keeping a journal as soon as I could manipulate a pencil, several months after the stroke. The journal became a tool for my survival; I used it to mark my progress, to ask the questions and articulate the fears I shared with no one else. My journal helped ground me in this strange new life where everything I had taken for granted—my body, my thoughts, the earth under my feet—had become shifting, unpredictable territory. The African-American writer Alice Walker once said that she writes the books she needs to read. Well, I was writing myself into understanding, into recovery of my self.

So initially I was not writing with a book in mind; in fact, I wanted to finish with this stroke thing and resume my life, which to me meant doing meaningful work in the world outside myself and my body. I was suspicious of what I considered to be people's morbid curiosity about the details of my stroke. But when I spoke about it publicly at the premiere of *Mile Zero*—the film I had begun before the stroke but did not complete until fourteen months after—the response changed my mind. People were more than just curious or sympathetic; they were hungry for information and talk about disability, loss, death. Strangers and friends told me stories about their father, their friend, their self, about disabilities they had never admitted to anyone, let alone discussed. A book could be useful.

I continued my daily handwritten journals. Soon there were volumes of flowered notebooks and miles of taped interviews with my husband Michael and our family, friends, and various health workers who played a role in our story. These conversations helped me retrieve memories of a time I was barely present. They also gave me a chance to tell each person what they had meant to me; in turn people told me how my illness had affected their lives.

Three years after my stroke, when I accompanied Michael on sabbatical in Boston, I sat down to write the book. But, again, life interfered with art: I found it too lonely to immerse myself in the painful past at the very moment when I felt ready to reenter the world. I shelved the book project, and even my journals became less regular as I started to figure out how to live as my new self. This meant getting to know other people with disabilities, and becoming part of the growing movement for disability rights.

When Michael and I finally settled in Vancouver, five and a half years after my stroke, I unpacked my journals and started work on what was to become the Canadian Broadcasting Corporation (CBC) radio series, "Bonnie and Gladys." Through the journals I retraced my odyssey and discovered connections and meanings that had been invisible to me while I was living it. Enough time had passed and I was finally ready to dive into the book.

Still, I knew I didn't want to be alone with all the memories and nightmares; I wanted company and the joy of creative collaboration that I had often experienced in my years as a documentary filmmaker with Canada's National Film Board. This seemed to be unusual in mainstream literary circles, where the writer works alone and hands the editor the resulting manuscript. Instead, I searched until I found the perfect collaborator, Persimmon Blackbridge.

Persimmon and I have much in common: We are both "crossovers" from other genres—I as a former filmmaker and Persimmon as a sculptor, video-maker and performance artist, as well as a writer of books. We are both feminists—though many would perceive us as polar opposites. As a member of the art collective Kiss & Tell, denounced as "that abhorrent lesbian show" in the Alberta legislature, Persimmon's work has been seized and banned by Canada Customs, while my anti-pornography film, *Not a Love Story*, got me labeled "Ms. Anti-Sex." But false dichotomies never got in the way of our respecting each other's work.

We are also both "disabled," though only my disabilities are visible. Persimmon has learning disabilities, which have given her a lifetime of practice in finding creative ways around unusual problems. She and I recognize each other's need for rest, time to search for the right word, or finish a thought. Persimmon is also a mental health system survivor, familiar with both terrors and labels.

Confident that I could trust Persimmon to help me tell my story, we sorted through the journals and tapes that I'd had transcribed onto computer disks. Persimmon then went home to her computer and organized this raw material—the film equivalent is "rushes"—a tedious and, to me, mind-boggling job.

While Persimmon was busy assembling and editing the material we had selected into a rough draft, I would be left with an "assignment" sheet full of her questions. They were designed to flesh out the details of the stories; weird questions like "What did the sheets feel like?"; "What did the physio smell like?" Smell?! I laughed at these questions, but as I sat outdoors with my notebook trying to answer them, the memories trickled, then flooded out. The physio smelled of coffee, and that reminded me of—well, you'll soon see.

When I thought I could remember no more, or procrastinated over a section, Persimmon suggested we "just talk about it" while I rested on my bed. Her careful listening made me feel safe enough to recover the worst horrors at last. We taped hours of additional memories, which Persimmon edited and cut into the narrative.

We got together regularly to trade goodies. I would give Persimmon new writing, and she would present me with an assembled morsel. The manuscript moved back and forth between us until we stopped knowing whose idea was whose. I would praise her for an apt phrase and Persimmon would say "Yes, it's from your journal." Our only arguments were to insist the other accept due credit. To say I "wrote" the book and Persimmon "edited" it would not acknowledge the reality of our collaborative process, or credit Persimmon's enormous sensitivity in drawing the story out of me, making elegant transitions between fragmented ideas, and devising literary solutions to ideological problems—not to mention walking my dog Lucy when I was too tired out, or the many hugs and laughs we shared.

~

As this book leaves our hands and goes out into the world, I am left with unresolved questions. The issue of language for describing disability nags at me. I choose the word "disabled" as the best of a bad lot. I dislike its negation of ability but I dislike even more those awkward euphemisms like "differently abled" or "physically challenged" that negate the daily physical struggle with which some of us live, as well as the discrimination we often face. Like the writer Nancy Mairs, I sometimes call myself a cripple, though that doesn't adequately describe my particular constellation of disabilities. Obviously, I cannot presume to label other people with such culturally-charged epithets.

I greatly prefer to name—and thereby reclaim—the truth, and believe the important thing is for each of us to name ourselves and tell our own stories. I'm more than a little pleased that, having been cast, I'm able to tell this one.

~ BONNIE SHERR KLEIN

Author's Note: In some instances names have been changed to protect privacy. In the vast majority of cases the names are real. The original Canadian edition of *Slow Dance* has been revised and updated for the United States edition.

STROKE ONE

❧ Prelude ❧

Journal: July 9, 1994

The wind has ripped through my notebook, losing my place and
interrupting the flow of words. I'm outside on a favorite park
bench, the one Michael calls my "office," feet resting on my
paisley electric scooter, Gladys, with Lucy, our golden retriever,
sprawled next to me. Behind me is blue sky busy with kites of
all shapes and tails, including a Star of David. And in their
midst, a Canadian flag outside the Coast Guard station. In front
of me is Vancouver's English Bay, full of pleasure boats, with
sailboats and kayaks scampering among them, and a few daring
swimmers. This is where I do my best writing. I still have
trouble being stuck indoors, after all my hospital incarcerations
and the isolation of Montreal winters where neither scooter nor
canes are safe on the icy streets.

Working at my desk would certainly be easier. It's 11:30 a.m. by the time I exercise, swim, eat breakfast and pack Gladys with my writing paraphernalia: sharp pencils, composition book, Persimmon's many questions and my scribbled notes, Lucy's doggy snacks and water bowl, my sunblock and sun hat, and today a *lunch* so I won't have to go back when I'm hungry. The only hitch is a bathroom for my frequent peeing, but there's a semi-accessible one (what I call half-assed-cessible) a short scoot away.

It strikes me that I needed these seven years to get to this place, this peace, where I feel safe to write. The memories are no longer a threat. Not only do I feel safe, but I'm excited. Each time I write I remember more. Even the painful memories are a strange pleasure, lost pieces of myself floating in on the tide.

❈ What I Did on My Summer Vacation ❈

Michael and I canoed the Missisquoi River, skinny-dipped in our homemade pond, and made love in the morning light. It was Monday, August 3, 1987. I think that was the day we pitched a tent—it was hot inside, and to sleep outdoors is a romantic notion that takes me back to my hippie days at Big Sur.

This was our first and last vacation alone in the Vermont cabin where we'd spent weekends and holidays with our children for the last ten years—the cabin that we'd finally decided to sell. The nest was emptying. Seth, now nineteen, would leave for the University of Toronto in the fall. Naomi, seventeen, had just graduated from high school. They were both back home in Montreal, with summer jobs.

I knew this marked a new phase of life and I felt bereft. I wasn't ready for the child-raising days to be over. Hard as it was to juggle the big F's of my life—family, filmmaking, and feminism—I wasn't ready to let go; I was only just beginning to get the hang of it.

But no kids meant long, lazy mornings in bed with my husband, a luxury I was prepared to appreciate. At home there was no such thing: Michael was Chief of Family Medicine at the Jewish General Hospital and a professor at McGill University. His life was crammed with patients and staff meetings and hospital politics and babies who insisted on being born in the middle of the night. Mine wasn't much different; if I wasn't off on a film shoot or buried in the editing room, I was at some emergency meeting to save Studio D, the feminist unit at the National Film Board where I was a staff film director.

Michael and I needed time to reconnect. On the surface, we were the Perfect Family, and I was the woman-who-had-it-all. I did, but not without a price, which was often my relationship with Michael. We had survived the tempestuous seventies when feminism rewrote the scripts of our lives. We had learned to balance very different and demanding and stressful professions, knowing we were there for each other to come home to. But a chronic source of conflict had to do with parenting Naomi. Michael responded to her painful and rebellious adolescence with anger. Although Naomi and I fought our own battles, I flinched at

Michael's impatience and sided with my female child, creating an impossible (and probably classic) familial knot. The last year had been one of the worst in our nearly twenty years of marriage.

It had been my worst year professionally as well. Studio D had turned down my most recent film proposal and I'd had to beg for private funding. I was furious at the rejection, but underneath the anger I was starting to doubt my worth as a filmmaker. Maybe at forty-six I was getting too old. Maybe documentary was passé. But filmmaking was all I knew—what on earth would I do with the rest of my life? Maybe on this vacation I would finally figure out what I wanted to be when I grew up.

$\sim$

Tuesday: the hottest day of the year. Michael and I set out early for a twenty-mile bicycle ride, all the way to Enosburg Falls. I loved riding, because or in spite of the fact that I only learned when Michael bought me a bicycle as a thirtieth birthday present. As an urban child my parents had forbidden me to learn to cycle. When Michael first tried to teach me, I promptly steered into a heavy chain blocking off a park road from automobile traffic. The chain caught me by the neck and threw me from the bike. Michael brought me home all bloody, sat me on our bathroom toilet and washed and stitched up my head. I continued to bicycle but it never became second nature to me, as it might have if I'd learned as a child.

On this hot day I was a worse rider than usual. I wavered over bumps and fell at a railroad crossing. My clothes clung to my sweaty body in uncomfortable places. My legs were two pieces of wood. I remember wondering, as I have frequently wondered while panting up the sides of various mountains: How much is too much? Where is the line between what's good for me and what's harmful? Will I know when to stop? Michael is a jock—he doesn't know the meaning of moderation; his idea of fun is to see how far he can push himself before he drops. My attitude had always been more laissez-faire, to do what I enjoy, like dancing and tennis, not earnest aerobics classes or stationary bicycles. But I knew I could no longer take my body for granted as I had my first forty years.

We turned back sooner than we'd planned, but we'd brought our tennis rackets knowing the town courts were on our way home. They were empty except for George, the town tennis pro. Too tempting. Michael trotted next door to the supermarket for a giant-sized sports drink and some bags of chips, vilely flavored with fake onion. I'd never had the sports drink before. It made me feel like a real athlete, even in my then pitiful condition.

So there I was on that morbidly hot day, exhausted but determined to keep up my end as we played two on one with George. I played embarrassingly badly. My face was purple, Michael told me later. Finally I quit and sat in the shade while Michael fought it out.

Afterwards, we bicycled the few miles back to our cabin. I spent the rest of the day hanging out in our bedroom, which was on the basement level dug into a hill, and so relatively cool. I had no appetite, but drank carton after carton of imported fruit juice. Clearly a case of heat prostration. Or maybe it was that disgusting bag of chips.

That night I spent stumbling between the bed and the bathroom. I couldn't walk without holding onto the walls. My legs were shaking and my guts were turning inside out. Michael slept soundly. I remember thinking, "This might be what dying feels like." But there was no reason for me to be dying, so I didn't wake him.

The next morning I called Muriel Duckworth and Kay Macpherson to say we would not be coming to float lanterns on Lake Memphramagog in memory of the bombing of Hiroshima. I was disappointed. Muriel and Kay are longtime peace activists, whom I met while making the film *Speaking Our Peace*. Muriel had become like a mother to me, a spiritual elder, her warmth embracing our whole family. Kay's sharp-edged humor brings my wilder flights of political idealism firmly down to earth. But this year, we would have no solemn, joyous ritual for peace. I was too sick.

By evening I was staggering when I walked; my tongue was thick and clumsy when I spoke, and I developed loud hiccups. These were clearly alarm signals for Michael. He didn't tell me what they could mean, but said that we probably shouldn't be stuck in the middle of the Vermont woods when we didn't know what was going on.

Michael: At 9 p.m., while giving you some tea, I noticed that your right eyelid was drooping, and your tongue deviated to the right. You were having some trouble swallowing due to simultaneous choking and hiccups. You had an unsteady gait, profound weakness, an up-going toe on the left with rhythmic oscillation in that ankle. These are brainstem and vestibular signs—not subtle.

I was upset. I knew where the trouble was located: all those signs are related to one small area in the brain stem where there's a series of nerve centers and tracks all crammed together. But I didn't know what the cause was. I certainly didn't think stroke—although the symptoms were stroke-like—because you were so healthy. There was no hypertension, no family history, no reason for it. I wanted to believe it was atypical migraine, or at worst food poisoning from the chips or fruit juice. Botulism affects those areas. For about an hour or so I was thinking of that.

But regardless of the cause, I was terrified because the nerve centers in that area are right next to the center that controls the respiratory system. All of those life-maintaining and control structures are right there within millimeters of each other. You could stop breathing.

Michael decided we had to get to an emergency room. Burlington, Vermont, was less than an hour away but he didn't know where the hospital was. He figured it would be better to drive like crazy the extra eighty kilometers to Montreal, than to get lost in Burlington in the middle of the night. He telephoned the Jewish General to say we were coming and then called the kids.

By this time it was midnight. Michael helped me up the few stone steps from the cabin and into the front of the station wagon. I wasn't sure I could handle the trip. I begged for some anti-nausea or sleeping medication, but he was afraid to give me any because of his unspoken worry that I might go into respiratory failure.

I traveled with plenty of throw-up bags, facecloths and tissue, with my head stuck out the window for the fresh night air. It was black as only the country night can be. The road was narrow and twisty through the mountains of Vermont. I don't remember any conversation except about how I was doing. Nothing hurt specifically—I was just all over miserable. I was even too miserable to be scared of Michael's driving, which must have been terrifying because he made what was usually a one hour and forty minute trip in fifty-five minutes. I suspect I dozed off, though I do remember the drama of whether we would have enough gas in our tank to take us all the way home.

I was worried about scaring Seth and Naomi. They were waiting for us; I don't know if they had been in bed before but now they were ready to go.

Seth: I can't remember who got the phone call. I guess it was fairly late. Dad said he was coming home to pick us up and then we were going to the hospital. I don't think we were worried at first. You and Dad came home, and we let Lucy out and helped Dad unpack the car to make room for us. Dad saved a couple of those juice containers to take to the hospital. He said you might have botulism. I didn't know what botulism was. The only thing that I knew from my first-aid training was that slurred speech was one of the symptoms of a stroke. I think I started to get worried at that point.

Naomi: I remember that night was really hot. The fan in my room was on and my boyfriend was over. The house looked the way it always looked when my parents were out of town: my stuff was all over the place; probably some alcohol and cigarette debris was around, and maybe even some evidence that my boyfriend and I had been sleeping in my parents' bed. Bad stuff. So when my brother told me that Dad had just called, that earlier reports of my mother's "stomach flu" were getting more serious and they were on their way home, my reaction was simple: Destroy the evidence. Clean the house.

By the time the car pulled up, the house was clean and the boyfriend was gone. My dad said that we should all go to the emergency room together. I came outside and saw my mother hanging out of the front seat. Her body was limp. I didn't remember sickness like this. Sickness that my dad couldn't fix with supplies from one of his medical bags: constipation, diarrhea, nausea; he would fix it. This he couldn't fix and I was scared.

I waited in the car, barely able to focus my eyes. I wanted to hurry up and get to the hospital and have them cure me. I expected a diagnosis and a quick solution. I never imagined that I wouldn't set foot in my home again for many months.

❧ Emergency Room ❧

The emergency room was a confused blur—too many people moving too fast in too little space. The last time I had been there was when my mother had some kind of infection related to her Alzheimer's. She spent several days in the corridor because there was no hospital bed available. There had been no room for a chair for visitors, and no privacy when she was examined.

JGH—Emergency Record: August 6
Subjective: 46 y/o WF. Previously healthy, no meds—2 day HX started with nausea, later blurred vision, diploplia, slurred speech. Drank imported peach juice.
Objective: Right ptosis, disconjugate gaze, double vision, discs sharp, sensation II intact, tongue to R, strength full in extremities, decreased sensation to light touch in L arm.
CT head: WNL
Diagnosis: Atypical migraine

I was seen by the emergency-room physician, a very young man who'd probably only been there a few months. He ordered a CAT (CT) scan. Michael was sure I had botulism and gave them the fruit-juice cartons to be tested.

Michael: I wasn't *sure* it was botulism. I just thought it was a possibility that should be checked. I didn't know what it was. I thought it might be vascular. But you weren't sick enough to have had a stroke in the usual sense of a hemispheric stroke.

At the same time it could have been atypical migraine. But you only had a little bit of headache. Everything was wrong. The tests showed nothing. By then it was 2 or 3 a.m. and you were stable and it wasn't progressing further. When you were lying down in bed in a safe environment you were your usual cheerful self.

I wanted to take you home. I didn't want you to be in the hospital. If you weren't in the hospital, of course you'd be OK.

Michael told the emergency-room physician that he would bring me back in the morning for more tests. The ER doctor thought I should stay. Michael insisted we go home. According to Naomi, Michael was bullying the poor guy, who was wildly outranked. Naomi rolled her eyes at me, long established shorthand for those "Father Knows Best" moments. I rolled mine back at her and we stifled our giggles.

Naomi: I stayed with my mother behind the curtain in the tiny examining cubicle. With my father arguing with the other doctor outside, we were suddenly relaxed. Something passed between us like a silent pact.

We'd been fighting since I was twelve. Our fights were less about actual transgressions than about my silence, my sullenness and, as my dad was always fond of putting it, my "refusal to be a part of this family."

But now there would be no more bull between Mom and me. We would stop fighting and be allies.

~

Meanwhile the ER doctor had the good judgment to call the attending neurologist, Joe Carlton. He gave me the first of what was to become hundreds of neurological exams.

Joe Carlton: When I heard that you had a problem and were in the emergency room, I sort of hoped against hope that it would turn out to be one of those minor things that just show up and then disappear, and you say in retrospect, Oh maybe it was just a migraine.

I had met you before at various JGH social occasions and we always talked. We shared many things that were difficult for me to share with my colleagues in medical circles. Literature, art, a certain way of looking at the world.

We kept saying we should get together for tennis doubles someday. I always hoped we would get to know each other better. But not in the emergency room.

I remember the sinking feeling in the pit of my stomach when I recognized that you had sustained clonus—involuntary shaking—in one of your ankles, which is a very serious finding usually associated with damage to the central nervous system. It could have been caused by a number of things, including a stroke.

Michael: I said to Joe Carlton, "Why don't I just take her home and I'll bring her into your office in the morning." He didn't hesitate, he just said, "Nonsense. We don't know what's going on here, but you're not taking her home. You be the husband and I'll be the doctor."

Michael relaxed then and so did I. Joe's presence changed everything. "Just wait," he said, "we'll be playing tennis soon." It was a joke, I knew it was a joke, but it sustained me for months. I repeated it over and over to myself: We had a date to play tennis. No matter how awful it was, Joe Carlton thought I would play tennis. And I knew Joe Carlton wouldn't lie.

They moved me to a cubicle to wait for the test results. I was feeling surprisingly calm considering the suddenness of this bolt from the blue and the apparent confusion surrounding it. I thought I was in good hands—the doctors could surely sort it out—and my family was closing around to protect me. Naomi held my hand. She had refused physical contact with me for years. But here in the hospital, it was truce time. I told her that I had finally decided what I wanted to be when I grew up: a witch. It sounded funny, even flaky. I didn't literally mean a practitioner of the rediscovered art of *wicca*, but I had been drawn to women who were exploring and expressing their spiritual authority.

Naomi: My mother was always saying things like that. She always wanted to be more of a hippie earth mother than she actually was and would often resolve to become something she simply was not, like a folksinger—an unfortunate aspiration considering she can neither sing nor play the guitar. The Joan Baez fantasy ran deep. It would resurface every few years and she would learn to play "Greensleeves" again.

Seth: We were in the ER for hours. There wasn't much to do. Hang out. Wait. Get a chocolate bar. Then suddenly you were being wheeled off to some other place where they had found you a bed and we had to leave. I'd never left anyone in a hospital before.

Patient Summary:
August 6 ... On exam patient showed horizontal nystagmus, worse on the right, deviation of the tongue to the right, right facial weakness, dysarthria, clonus of the left ankle, and decreased pain sensation in the left foot and left leg and thorax to the T2 level ... Proposed diagnosis of right medullary ischemia (local lack of oxygen to right medulla—cause not yet established).

❃ Surgical Intensive Care Unit ❃

The surgical ICU was one big open room, with people attached to machines in curtained-off cubicles and other people walking around with clipboards. I knew and disliked the surgeon-in-charge. He had once threatened to report a friend of mine for child abuse, for breast-feeding her baby while she had mastitis and a breast abscess, which Michael had assured me is harmless to the baby and good treatment for the abscess.

The surgeon came by in the morning, a herd of medical students in his wake. The thin muslin curtains around my bed were drawn, but I recognized his voice. He stood just outside my cubicle and read my chart.

"The precise diagnosis is not clear," he told his entourage, "but the bottom line is, it can't be anything good."

I don't remember if I tried to say something. My voice was weak, but I could still talk at that point. I was furious that he would talk about me as if I wasn't there.

I was still too ignorant about the grim diagnostic possibilities to be scared.

My next visitor couldn't have been more different. My personal family practitioner, Irene Kupferszmidt, had escaped the Nazi invasion of Poland when she was nineteen. She was tough enough to stand up to my doctor husband when necessary, but they had great mutual respect.

Irene Kupferszmidt: It was Thursday morning, I was sitting on the chair at the hairdresser's. My son Henry was going to be married that night, a small family wedding, and I was getting myself fixed up. And just as the hairdresser was pouring the water over my head, my secretary called to say you were in hospital. I jumped up and ran—left the hairdresser standing there with her mouth open!—and arrived at the hospital looking like a crazy lady with a babushka on her head, not a respectable doctor.

I looked at you and thought, it could be anything. Maybe some viral thing, one of those sicknesses that we never diagnose that simply disappear. That was denial maybe.

My first thought when I saw her was, if Irene who is a model of impeccable taste and coiffure rushes in looking like this, I must really be sick. That was the moment I knew this could be serious.

Consultation report—August 6
Dr. Carlton: Possible vertebrobasilar ischemia. R/o evolving brain-stem infarct. R/o viral encephalomyelitis.
Dr. Black: Right 7th and possibly 8th palsy that suggests it is secondary to a medullary infarct. Recommend feeding tube.
Dr. Libman: Likely an ischemic lesion of the right medulla. Doubt inflammatory disease.
Dr. Wise: Possible right medullary syndrome with central Horners and divergence insufficiency horizontal and vertical nystagmus involving the 7th cranial nerve. Possible post viral demyelanating disease?
CT scan—negative
echocardiogram—negative
LP—negative
arteriogram—negative

I spent the whole of that afternoon lying on a tall bed and being wheeled through various departments, receiving test after test. I just lay there while they whisked me about and did things to me.

I remember nervously waiting in a corridor for the arteriogram, a diagnostic procedure where they stick a needle into one of your arteries and inject a dye that makes all the blood vessels in your head visible by x-ray. The doctor in charge told me that there was a very slight risk associated with it—in a very few cases the dye can cause spasms in the blood vessels, leading to a stroke—so he was obliged to ask me to sign a consent form. Michael told me it was OK; he knew and trusted this guy. But I wondered what I would have done if I had been alone. How could I possibly assess the risks this stranger proposed I take? If I was feeling overwhelmed, what about someone who doesn't happen to have a physician in the family?

I was poked and prodded by everyone from medical students who looked all of seventeen, to all the department chiefs, who each looked at whatever part of the "elephant" they specialized in, and diagnosed accordingly. The number one diagnosis was stroke. This was the first time I had heard them use the word stroke. I couldn't take it in. It seemed unreal—only old people have strokes.

Michael explained to me that there were many kinds of stroke, and that it was important to know whether mine was caused by a clot or a bleed. If it was a clot, anticoagulants would be used, but if it was a bleed, anticoagulants could make it worse. The first CT scan showed no evidence of bleed, so they put me on an anticoagulant named Heparin.

~

I was too exhausted from two nights of sleeplessness to sort out, let alone participate in, the medical arguments about my diagnosis and treatment. Instead, I worried about my current film. *Mile Zero* documented the cross-Canada high school speaking tour of four students, including my son Seth, from SAGE (Students Against Global Extermination). They believed that teenagers could work towards peace rather than accept the fear and hopelessness that affected many young people in those Cold War years. After months of preparation they set off on a fifty-city tour, joined from time to time by a film crew and an anxious mother/director.

Both the tour and the shooting had been finished in May but the long, demanding process of editing had only started. What would happen to the film if I had to stay in the hospital for a few weeks, or even a month? We would get hopelessly behind schedule. On our slim budget, we had hired Sidonie Kerr, a freelance film editor whose work I admired, on a six-month contract with the assumption that I would be there to work full time beside her. I didn't want to lose her.

Sidonie Kerr: I had just started working with you a month before, as the editor of *Mile Zero*. I hardly knew you, and I felt—as I always do as editor—a certain guardedness. We had planned simultaneous vacations so we wouldn't lose time from the film. And then my son Robbie phoned me with the news that you were in the hospital.

On my return I found a note dictated by you, written by Naomi. It said how badly you felt for me coming home to an illness, but that you trusted me to forge ahead without you. I think that was the beginning of my real commitment. What was just an interesting assignment became totally involving. It was a decision that wasn't even a decision. I was going to do whatever it took to help you finish your film.

❈ Neurological Intensive Care Unit ❈

The next day I was transferred yet again, this time to the neurological ICU. Late that night I received my first ever acupuncture treatment.

Bernard Coté had treated Michael's back pain with acupuncture on and off for the past three years. Michael had attended the birth of Bernard's last child. Sometimes they had worked together, as doctor and acupuncturist, assisting difficult births. They had become colleagues and close friends: an odd couple, given most Western physicians' professional chauvinism.

When Michael told me Bernard was going to give me a treatment, I was surprised. Although I knew acupuncture was useful for other conditions—smoking, muscle and joint pain, insomnia—I never associated it with serious illness. Bernard had just returned from Tianjin, where, it turned out, he had been studying acupuncture techniques for stroke patients. In China, acupuncture is an integrated part of hospital medicine, and the primary treatment for stroke, but Bernard had never expected to use his new skills in an acute-care setting in high-tech Montreal. Because Bernard wasn't an MD, Michael had to obtain special permission from the Medical Director.

I was delighted to see Bernard. When he came into my dingy cubicle, he was sweet as always, saying "What a silly thing to happen on your vacation." Bernard and Michael had plotted it all out. Bernard wanted to use moxabustion, which involves burning a bundle of herbs (moxa) to intensify the effect of the needles. The hospital room was equipped with a hair-trigger smoke detector and sprinkler system which Bernard did not think would enhance the treatment. Michael climbed on my bed and dismantled the smoke detector, while I, good girl that I am, froze in fear that a passing nurse would catch us. What did I think would happen? We would be expelled? Yelled at? Fired? The fact that moxa smells a lot like pot didn't help my fears, but there was also something delicious about being naughty.

I was a bit apprehensive—I was afraid of needles. I had always chosen chiropractic or massage for my own low-back spasms; I couldn't imagine how needles could ever relax anything. And what if Bernard "missed" and made my condition worse?

Bernard examined me by taking my pulse, first in one wrist then in the other. He looked at my tongue and asked me to breathe in and out. After swabbing my skin with alcohol at the first acupuncture point, he inserted a thin steel needle. I looked away. I don't remember the exact points he punctured—I think there were needles in my ears and legs and in my tongue, which felt weird. Some needles were shallow, just through my skin. Others were up to an inch and a half deep. Mostly they stayed in for ten minutes or so. Every now and then he would twiddle them a few times. Some needles were like a jolt of electricity, a deep tingling or a dull ache. Others wouldn't feel like much at first and then *thong!*—a big hand tightening like a fist. Others felt like nothing at all, and I was afraid to turn over without asking Bernard if it was OK, in case these phantom needles were still in me.

I remember a great peace after the treatment, followed by a burst of energy. My speech was clearer and I was choking less. Michael says my right eyelid lifted dramatically—a good sign. We all committed to continue. Bernard would come twice a day while I needed it, which I didn't imagine would be long. He wouldn't let us speak of payment.

I fell asleep calm and optimistic. Being in the hospital seemed like an interesting interlude, a strange country I would pass through like a tourist, curious and unaltered.

August 7
00:00   Received pt awake in bed.
         Heparin drip at 22 cc/hr. infusing well in forearm.
09:15   Neurology: Pt claims speech is more difficult. Diplopia
         more prominent.
         Pt complains swallowing more difficult.
10:30   Infusion dye injected.

CT scan, shows hemorrhagic infarction, right medulla.
Stop Heparin drip, D5W to KVO.

Joe Carlton: The next day you seemed a bit worse. We got another CT scan which looked more closely at the posterior of the brain stem, and this time there was evidence of a bleed: a hemorrhage in the medulla. Which meant that, in retrospect, an anticoagulant like Heparin had been a very bad choice. It was a minor miracle that your condition did not deteriorate more. That was my first heavy piece of baggage.

The cold intimacy of the hospital notes. I have become Pt (patient) instead of a person with a name. Pt complains . . . Pt claims . . . Pt refuses . . . I watch myself sink into the institutional limbo: no day, no night, just rounds and meds and tests and restless snatches of sleep.

~

I don't know where to start, why I remember so poorly. My best guess is that my body and mind were too sleepy. I must have been a bizarre sight with all the equipment I was fastened to: IV lines, suction tube, feeding tube. I got so used to the IV needle I didn't even know it was in, except when the tubing and the stand got in the way—tangled up with other tubes or the cord on the earphones I wore for music.

I was given a patch to wear on my left eye to alleviate my double vision and the dizziness it caused. I didn't recognize myself in the short hospital gown, ugly white anti-embolic stockings and eye patch.

The tube was a plastic suction tube used to remove the

constant mucus and saliva from my mouth. I never realized how often you have to swallow until I couldn't do it. I felt as if I would be choked or drowned by my own secretions. My lips were parched from the suctioning.

In the bathroom, the nurse catheterized me "in-and-out" because I had trouble voiding. In-and-out means that the tube is removed after the bladder is emptied, unlike with an in-dwelling catheter, which I had later. I remember being relieved that it didn't hurt much, although that would vary with the nurse; some were gentler than others. I remember being impressed that urine could be removed in this impersonal way. After a few days I was able to pee by myself again, but by then I had developed a urinary tract infection.

I had a few toys that Bernard gave me. One was like a little wooden rolling pin with spikes, to roll around with my foot for stimulation and practice in control and intention. He also brought a few small, Chinese wooden balls, apricot size. You could see the grain in the unfinished wood—it smelled like cedar. He suggested I squeeze them in my hand as often as I could. As with the acupuncture, I didn't really understand, but I did it all faithfully. I liked having something active to do to care for myself. The medical doctors were into diagnosing; if they asked me how I was feeling, it was only as a test to figure out what was going on, not to address the symptom and provide a practical way to cope with it. The Chinese balls also gave me the feeling that somebody had been here before me, that this was a very old, very simple technique for a fairly common problem.

The hospital was stifling in this typical Montreal mid-August. It smelled like piss and industrial strength cleanser. It was also very dry, and I felt as if I couldn't breathe. Michael brought a small humidifier from home and Irene Kupferszmidt brought me mineral water in a beautiful spray-mist bottle. I had never used a mister before. It made me feel like an exotic plant, and I used it constantly. I don't know how Irene knew, but it was exactly what I needed.

The nurses often rubbed my back with something like alcohol. I think it was supposed to prevent bedsores or help me relax so I could sleep. There are many nurses' notes about sleeplessness. I don't think there was a specific reason, though one note says "anxious." Probably it was everything that was going on in my traumatized brain. I was fatigued yet I couldn't sleep, a vicious cycle. It was better when I had late-night acupuncture treatments. The other big help was music. I became addicted to music. I always wore earphones. Michael brought all our favorite tapes and friends made me personal tapes of music they loved: Yiddish classics from Adrianne Sklar, Sidonie's *La Traviata,* flute meditations from Kathleen Shannon, my longtime boss at Studio D.

During these first few days in the hospital, I felt strangely peaceful. Whatever was going on in my body was clearly out of my control. I didn't believe in any Divine Plan, but neither did I believe this was a random accident. I didn't ask "why me?" but felt rather that it was my turn—I who had always been so privileged and lucky.

Irene Kupferszmidt: Over the next week I was in and out. You were getting a little better every day but you were still very tired. Your friends kept walking into your room, especially ones who worked with Michael. I resent very much that custom. I feel it's barbaric. They make a social event out of illness and they disturb the patient. So I put up a sign for you after the first few days. *No visitors—and that includes Michael's friends in white coats.*

There were so many doctors, high-powered specialists. I would think to go see you but then I'd tell myself I have nothing positive at this moment to tell her. But when you were asleep, I sometimes came in and looked at you. I tiptoed because you were having trouble sleeping and I didn't want to disturb you out of your rest.

Naomi: The summer of the stroke, I had a job doing clerical work at the JGH emergency room. When my mother got sick, I went into my boss's office and told him that I was quitting. He was very understanding. I remember exactly what he said: "The recovery is going to be very long and very slow. It could take months, even years. But there is one thing about stroke: It only gets better. It doesn't get worse." I was very moved by what he said and very excited. I told my mother: "Dr. Afilalo says that it will only get better. It can't get worse." I repeated that phrase to myself over and over again like a mantra. "It can only get better. It can't get worse."

Michael: It wasn't as terrible as it might have been. You were alive and your functions were coming back. You were able to use the toilet, to transfer from the bed to the wheelchair. But you were still very sick.

I was the director of Herzl at the time, the family medicine outpatient center at the JGH. But I stopped working. I stopped doing the office practice; I stopped doing administration. There were sixty people on my staff at Herzl, plus 100 doctors in the Department of Family Medicine that I was responsible for. And they covered for me. They did my work. They looked after me. The nurses, the doctors, people were with me constantly. Those were the people I cried with.

All I did was deliver babies.

I remember each one.

I practice a sort of midwifery, helping people in what is essentially a normal process. Childbirth isn't an illness, and it's rarely life threatening. I was percolating between your room on the third floor and the delivery suite on the fifth floor, selfishly using attendance at birth as psychotherapy: a break from my concerns for you.

What I couldn't do while you were sick was sit still and listen to somebody's minor ailments, which of course to them are major. And I couldn't deal with administrative work at all. I had no patience for it.

That was one of the consequences of your illness, which is not necessarily beneficial. I had zero tolerance for bull.

Naomi and Seth visited frequently, but most of my friends were held at bay by Irene's sign. They phoned or sent cards instead. Shul friends said prayers, and Studio D pagans performed rituals on Mount Royal. As my energy improved, I started to make a few exceptions to Irene's rule. Ron Aigen, the rabbi at our synagogue came every day. I assumed that he was just dropping by while giving "spiritual succor" to older people in the hospital. Then I realized *I* was sick and he was visiting *me*.

Rabbi Ron was more important to me than either of us would have anticipated. When I told him several years later how much his presence had meant to me, he revealed that he had felt hesitant to impose himself. He did not want to take advantage of my situation to suddenly bring me religion.

Ron connected me to the piece of my life which I felt had been short-changed in my relationship with Michael, the son of left-wing atheists. It's a piece of my childhood, my upbringing in a traditional Jewish family. Ron is low-key, very warm and calm. He fits no stereotype of a rabbi, which is why Michael likes him as much as I do. He has nothing to "sell." His spiritual leadership is by unpretentious example. I always loved going to shul to watch him pray. He exudes a quiet joy.

Ron told me that he had said a Healing Prayer for me in shul—the prayer said at the high point of the Shabbat, when the Ark is open and the Torah is being read. It asks that the One who blessed our ancestors (traditionally it names our forefathers, Abraham, Isaac, and Jacob, but our Reconstructionist synagogue adds our foremothers, Sarah, Rebecca, Rachel, and Leah) bless and completely heal who-ever is sick, in my case Bat-Shira, Daughter of Song, the Hebrew name I made up for myself when I was a teenager at a Hebrew-speaking summer camp.

Though he seemed relaxed on his visits, Ron later told me he was devastated by my stroke. "I did a lot of pastoral work with older congregants, but you were close to my age, a peer and a friend. This wasn't supposed to happen to you."

I was in the neurological ICU for four days. Most of the other patients were too sick to talk, but the staff was like one big dysfunctional family—intimate and inescapable. It had its good side, however. There was one orderly named Georgio with a mustache and an accent that was Greek or maybe Italian. He treated me with old-world gallantry and made me feel like a queen. I learned to stand (with help), lock my knees and pivot from the bed to the wheelchair, or the wheelchair to the toilet, a move which Georgio translated into a dance. He would say, "Want to dance with me?" And then he'd lift me and sing, "Now we dance" as he helped pivot me onto the toilet. I always looked forward to his shifts. He made something that everyone else treated as a real chore into fun, as though our moments together were pleasant for him as well as for me.

There was another orderly whom I thought of as The Giant. He was bald like Telly Savales and very tall. He didn't talk much, but he would notice when my tray table had been left out of reach, and push it back without being asked.

Suzi Scott was my favorite nurse. Seth and Naomi already knew her as a familiar face, the mother of children with whom they'd gone to school. The staff tended to ignore Naomi unless she did something they didn't like. She had already argued with a few nurses when she'd taped get-well cards up on the glass wall that separated my little alcove from the main ward. But Suzi welcomed Naomi, teaching her nursing tricks like shampooing my hair in a bedpan.

Naomi: Suzi Scott was like an angel, a loving human being who swooped in and saved us from the heartless, machine-like, nurse androids. She loved us, she gushed all over us. The truth is that if I met Suzi Scott under any other circumstances, I probably would have hated her. I couldn't stand saccharine, manic people, who touch you too much and love you too much and look too deeply into your eyes. When everything is all right, you can afford to hate really nice people. When things suck, they really come in handy.

August 8, 13:40. Dietitians Note:
Pt was receiving 1/2 strength concentrated liquid nutritional supplement at 50 mL/hr. via Dobhoff and had diarrhea.

Recommend 1/4 strength concentrated liquid nutritional supplement at 50 mL/hr. for today. Pt has also tried semisolids such as custard this afternoon but she claims she's not up to it yet.

Pt claims to be able to swallow w/o any discomfort but says that "One muscle at the end of swallowing won't do what I want it to do."

I had diarrhea from the supplement, an enriched formula that I was fed by nose tube four times a day. It was a thick, yellowish liquid which came in a blue plastic bottle. My Mom had been fed the same stuff when she was hospitalized. The smell of it nauseated me. I did not want to be my mother lying helpless in a hospital bed, fed through a tube, the same smell, drifting further and further into absence.

The high point of my day was Joe Carlton's rounds. I could count on him to tell me what was going on. He would sit on my bed in the evening, looking exhausted. I knew his wife and kids were waiting for him, as I had so often waited for Michael, impatient with all those needy people stealing his time from me. But now I felt a desperate dependence. I wanted Joe to stay, to talk, to explain things over and over. My body ached, I was sleeping badly, I was sick of being strong. What I needed from Joe was just the sound of his voice, tired and calm, soothing me with honest, uncertain explanations.

August 10

04:35   Pt states Dobhoff tube fell out—MD notified—Pt hungry. Two small teaspoons Jell-O—Pt spit it out.
08:00   Dobhoff tube inserted by resident.
14:00   Pt refused to sit up in chair. Stated she is too tired.
14:15   Pt transferred to Neuro High-Care.

❧ Neurological High-Care Unit ❧

When our longtime housekeeper, Meena Williams, came to visit, I had graduated to the Neuro High-Care Unit. High-Care was a big room right across from the nurses' station, with a sliding glass door so the nurses could keep an eye on us and still do their endless paperwork. There were four beds; I was next to the window, though I was too sick to look out.

Meena Williams: There were no visitors allowed when you were first sick. So I waited until it was time. When I came in, you grabbed for my hand and we held onto each other. You asked me if I would go and visit your mother for you because you didn't want her to feel she had been abandoned. And I was happy to do it. Your mom and I always got along very well.

By that time, her memory had begun fading and she couldn't remember everybody. I would say to her, "Bonnie sends her love and she'll be back soon." And she'd just look. I felt she recognized me because she smiled. I would brush her hair, trim her nails. I could see there was some satisfaction. But not being able to move around, after how active she used to be—I think that was hard on her. But comes the time, you know.

I had all the possessions that constituted my world arranged around me: cards and mobiles, a small box of hospital tissue, my tape player, the apricot lip balm that Studio D friends gave me in a basket of treats from the Body Shop. Next to my bed was the ubiquitous sliding hospital tray table on wheels and a little metal cabinet. There were plants on the skimpy windowsill until the nurse Naomi called The Hun confiscated them because they were "unhealthy."

In the NICU, my cubicle had been in an alcove away from the other patients. High-Care was my first real experience of ward life. It was very quiet as all three of my roommates were in deep comas. I felt like I was in a roomful of corpses.

The woman in the bed next to mine was named Patricia. She had been in a freak car accident where a construction crane fell through her front windshield crushing her skull. She'd been in a coma for six months. She was totally unresponsive. Her husband, J.P., would sit by her bedside every day for hours. He just sat there and spoke to her in an endless mumbled litany: *"Patricia je t'aime. Ma belle fille, ma p'tite, ma cherie . . ."* I would lie there thinking, what an utter waste of time. As far as I could tell she was gone—dead. But J.P. kept on and on. He never gave up.

I was thrilled when after one day in High-Care, I was moved to a private room.

⇌ Interlude: Mom ⇌

Journal: July 30, 1994

I am on the ferry en route to Gabriola Island off the coast of British Columbia for the long weekend. The heat wave has finally broken—I am amazed at how well I endured it this time. The ferry is one of my favorite places to work. I feel so privileged to be writing here among the fishing eagles.

Getting ready for this trip was miserable. Some of my behavior reminds me of my mother. Mechanical incompetence. Losing my eyeglasses. Having to repeat the plan several times so I'll be sure to remember everything. Needing to pee, worrying about when, where. Needing routines, rigidity. Writing notes to myself, lists like Mom had all over the house.

Sometimes I feel that Michael is ordering me around, talking down to me as if I were a child. "Go to the bathroom now because there's a toilet." "Lie down and take a rest; you're tired." Is it fear I see in Michael's eyes, when he flares with impatience at my constant needs?

Mom. Vacant, trapped. Still but not serene. "Practical"

clothes: cheap synthetic housedresses, Velcro shoes, elasticized waists; easy to put on, easy to clean. She used to be such
a fashion plate. But always messy, like me. Each of us used to
get stains on the best-silked tips of our boobs—but that pre-
dates both Alzheimer's and strokes.

I don't want to be her. Her gnarled hands. Her bunioned
feet. Her toothless smile. Her breastless chest. Her body like a
lost, frail little boy, not the Russian matriarch who once was my
mother. I worked so hard to hold onto the memory of my
mother, how she was. I tried for so long to make her remember.

She died in slow motion over many years. Years of misplac-
ing keys and glasses, then accusing various housecleaners of
stealing them. Making endless lists of things to do and having
to ask the same questions over and over. Piling furniture to bar-
ricade the apartment door against the imaginary man who had
stolen her key and was trying to break in. Michael finally insist-
ing that she give up her driver's license.

In 1980, my sister Razelle called me back from Michael's
sabbatical in England when Mom was diagnosed with breast
cancer for the second time. Her first breast had been removed a
year after my father died, in 1968. The second surgery acceler-
ated her decline, I think. I had to accompany her to each
procedure, to explain and reexplain what was happening, the
implication of each finding and each decision. It was the first
clear sign I had of her childlike passivity, this woman who had
been so sharp and questioning, such a fighter, all her life.

Several years later came the move to Montreal, the painful
months of living with us, the final euphemistic "foster home"
when she became too paranoid to be left even with Meena.

I felt guilty on days I didn't stop to visit her on my way home from work. I thought she had nothing to do but wait for the joy of my meager visits. "Where have you been?" she'd say. "It's been a long time." Even when it was yesterday. And then painful goodbyes after pleasant visits. "Are you leaving so soon? I think I'll go with you." I begged her with all my rationality not to make me feel guilty about living my life as she had always taught me: "Your husband and children come before everyone else."

But soon she just greeted me with a big focusless smile and said, "What a nice surprise. I wasn't expecting you," in her most sociable, sweet manner. She would show me off to her housemates, remembering neither their names nor mine. I learned to say, "Hi Mother dear, it's your daughter Bonnie," to spare her the shame of not knowing. She would brag about what a thoughtful, wonderful daughter she had, how I took such good care of her. She used to expect Dad too, forgetting he'd died years ago. Then one day she no longer remembered him, not even when I pushed it. It was as if their long life together had never happened.

And just as I was getting used to the absent, childlike sweetness and obsequious gratitude, my mother forgot me entirely.

Sometimes I would think that she was purposely not recognizing me, to punish me. That she was angry I'd abandoned her, contrary to the wish she'd expressed in earlier years never to be "stuck away in an institution." As she had abandoned the aunt who helped raise her after her mother died and her father deserted her. Tanta lived with us throughout her later years. I was

too young to understand what became wrong with her, but I remember my mother shopping for the least awful nursing home
and visiting her there. I remember my mother's guilt that she
couldn't conduct her real estate business and raise her own
family and still care for Tanta.

As I write, I wonder about me and my children. What do
you do with a mother who can no longer care for herself? What
do you do?

❈ A Room of My Own ❈

Moving into a private room meant I was getting better. I no
longer needed constant nursing care. After five days in the
hospital, I still couldn't walk unassisted or swallow, but I
could now stand and transfer to the toilet by myself, and
the rest would surely come in another week or two. The
nurse showed me how my new bed could be raised and
lowered and tilted at many different angles; the head, the
middle, and the foot all moved separately, but I couldn't
begin to sort it out. She showed me the call button to buzz
for emergencies since I was no longer right in front of the
nursing station. She clipped the cord to my heavy pillow
case, which smelled of disinfectant and had Jewish General
Hospital stamped on its hem, and placed the button itself
in my hand. I was alone and secure.

No sooner had I settled in when a man in pajamas wandered in, noisily demanding a cigarette and matches. I tried
to refuse him politely but he insisted, pacing my room and

shouting. I was frightened and pushed the buzzer. The nurse came in no great hurry. She thought it was funny and shooed him away with no word to me.

Michael: We were in bed watching television the first night in your private room. I had a sore back, and your bed was definitely the place to be. I was frequently in bed with you. We would hold hands and talk, or we would watch television. I also read to you. But this one night we were watching the World Series. I can't remember who was playing, or how interested we were.

And then, I don't know how it started but we were making love. We didn't actually have intercourse. But we were involved in very heavy petting. I remember feeling that it wouldn't be harmful. In the ICU, you were attached to too many pieces of equipment. But now we could, and we had a mutual need. You had an orgasm. It was good for both of us, even in the hospital.

Though you were getting better, you were still very sick. You moved differently. And underneath it all there was this frightening feeling that it might be the last orgasm for a long time.

I was totally turned on and totally embarrassed. I didn't think this kind of thing was allowed in a hospital. Somebody could walk in and there's the Chief of Family Medicine in bed with a patient. I had such a mix of reactions. Part of me was thinking: What kind of sex maniac is he? Is he trying to deny what's happening? Is he so desperate that I be well? Is he trying to prove our life will be the same?

But past all embarrassment and analysis, Michael

touched me. I could feel that he loved me. This body that was poked and prodded by daily strangers like a lump of meat was still lovable. He made me feel that this body was still mine.

August 11
23:30   Husband still visiting.
         Pt anxious, trying to sleep. Awaking easily.

Over the next few days, Naomi de-institutionalized my new room. She had always been into nesting, while I was as oblivious to my surroundings as I was to my body. It was one of our ongoing tensions; I thought she was too concerned with appearances and she thought I was an unfeminine slob. But even I could appreciate the transformation she wrought in that hospital room. The walls ran riot with art cards, nature cards, seriously drippy get-well cards, corny chicken soup joke cards. And every few days a new note from my Studio D colleague and good friend Terre Nash:

> *August 12*
> *Dearest Darling Bonnie, Enclosed is an item of extreme importance—a Nancy Reagan NOSE-MASK. Whenever you get tired of having people around or of tests being administered, etc., just put on the nose-mask. It scares the shit out of people and they will go away. . . .*
> *love, Terre*

My oldest friend and Studio D office mate, Dorothy Hénaut, sent a different painting almost every day: orange day lilies; endless fields of bright apple green; a landscape with purple cows. The hospital staff would come by just to see the new art. Seth brought a radio. He wanted me to be able to listen to "Morningside" and public affairs programs, to have some connection to the outside world. Naomi brought back my banned plants and I kept receiving new ones, which soon took over the room.

One of my most treasured presents was a shoebox filled with the tiniest paper cranes, which had been folded by Muriel Duckworth's granddaughter Danielle. Cranes are a Japanese symbol of healing which came to be a peace symbol through the story of Sedako, an eleven-year-old runner who got cancer as a result of radiation poisoning from the bombing of Hiroshima. Legend tells that if a thousand paper cranes are folded for someone, they will be healed. Sedako folded 640 before she died. Her classmates completed the thousand, and now children from all over the world place necklaces of paper cranes on a sculpture of Sedako in Hiroshima. A clip of Muriel Duckworth placing cranes from the schoolchildren of Halifax at the feet of that sculpture is one of my favorite images in *Speaking Our Peace.*

August 12

07:30   up in commode x 2—cloudy foul-smelling urine
         and diarrhea
         Mobility: Sat x 20 minutes by side of bed. C/o tiredness.

12:00   Magnetic Resonance Imaging requested. (Dr. Carlton)
         Radiologist thought MRI not urgent. Over next 2 weeks

should be OK if pt clinically stable. MRI should be done
before next CT.

R/o Cavernous angioma.

Naomi: When you heard about the MRI, you said, "Why
more tests—don't we know I had a stroke?"
Joe said, "Just a few more, for my peace of mind."
You asked, "Is it claustrophobic?"
Joe said, "Well, you have to lie inside the machine, per-
fectly still, for forty-five minutes."
You said, "Do I have to?"
Joe said, "I'm going on vacation; we'll talk about it when I
get back."

I knew there was still disagreement among the JGH doctors, but I was ready to accept the diagnosis of stroke. I
didn't understand why we needed to know more. I didn't
realize that many things can cause a stroke—it could be
cancer, or a blood clot, or a hemorrhage that might bleed
again. I didn't realize that depending on the cause, the treatment might be different. As far as I was concerned, whatever
had happened was now over and done with, and I was ready
to move on to rehabilitation so I could resume my life.

I was put in the hands of the Stroke Team, a trio of
women, only one of whom seemed to have a clear and practical function: the physiotherapist, Iolanda Zompa. She had
dark curly hair, mischievous eyes, and smelled fragrantly
of strong coffee. She seemed confident and calm, as if she
had seen many people in my condition. She was the first in
a long line of physio cheerleaders with whom I fell in love.

Her attitude was "I know you can do it." And when I did, she would say, "*Yesss*, Bonnie, you did it!"

The big job of the Stroke Team was to teach me to swallow. Iolanda and the speech therapist both worked on that. They would feed me brightly colored popsicles, then check the tube to see if the color of the secretions I was choking on matched the popsicles. If not, I was swallowing.

August 17

All exercises to be carried out in the presence of a nurse—
10 consecutive reps, 3x daily.

(1) Phonation

    (a) ah

    (b) ah-cha

    (c) click

(2) Tongue movements

    (a) tip of tongue along roof of mouth

    (b) tip of tongue along floor of mouth

    (c) protrude tongue

    (d) elevate tongue to nose, to chin

    (e) lick lips

    (f) push tip of tongue against tongue depressor

(3) Cough

(4) Take small sips, with a straw, of a liquid at mealtime. A minimum of 2 oz. to be ingested per meal.

Sip, swish fluid around in mouth for a moment & swallow, then swallow again, immediately (i.e. 2 swallows).

(5) Suckle ice cubes, aggressively, & swallow water (2 swallows).

(6) Chew gum (in presence of family or nurse). (Please note: spit out when too soft.)

(7) Chew on tongue depressor & swallow saliva.

I did my swallowing exercises religiously. I did physical exercises too: leg raises and kicks in bed or up in the chair. Iolanda brought a walker, so I could go to the toilet by myself. It was the kind with no wheels—just a folding frame that gave four-point support when it was open. It gave me enough stability to walk a bit if Iolanda held me too, either by the nape of the neck or by the waist, like I may have held Seth and Naomi when they were first learning to walk. I had to lift the frame and put it down for each step, advancing it and then moving towards it. My mother was using a walker in the foster home. How would the kids feel seeing me look like their grandmother?

Naomi: One day I came for a visit. You were in the hall with the physio and she was helping you walk, like you used to help your mom. So I stopped in the nursing station to talk to Dad and Joe Carlton and some other people I knew. There was glass across the whole front of the nursing station, so you could see everywhere. I guess it was the first time that I was watching you rather than being with you and talking to you. Usually if I could see you walk, I would be right there helping you. But in this situation I was just sort of observing you through the glass, from a distance. As I watched, the room started spinning, and I said "Dad, I really don't feel well." Then I fainted. He lay me down and took my pulse, and I was out for two seconds or something. It was really weird. There was no warning. There was no emotional thing attached to it. It was a purely physical response.

Iolanda and I worked hard. The notes indicate that I

was improving a bit every day. We gradually increased the distance I could walk. I was hesitant and bumbling, but I remember when I finally walked from my room to the nurses' station. Joe Carlton and the nurses burst into spontaneous applause, and I collapsed with exhaustion.

There was the old and continuing question of how much to push, when is enough and when am I being lazy or indulgent? Would one more step make me too tired? Was it good for me? I still feel guilty when I read in the nurses' notes: "Pt c/o [complains of] being fatigued, refused to sit in chair."

Despite my daily confrontations with the limits of my body, I still felt that the stroke wasn't real. It didn't touch me. It was something weird, and temporary, that had happened to my body but not to *me*. I was the same person I'd always been and we were all working hard, so everything would of course turn out all right.

Since we didn't know the cause of my stroke, I assumed it was stress. The idea that I'd somehow brought it on myself was hard to shake. Maybe I'd been living too long in the fast lane and was now paying the price for trying to have it all. Or perhaps I was "stroked out" by my work environment, fighting so hard to make a film in which I believed, in an institution which did not seem to believe in me.

∽

Mile Zero had certainly been stressful. Without NFB sponsorship, I had sought the fund-raising help of an independent co-producer, Irene Angelico. We hustled for private funds, and did the first shoot using my personal credit card for travel costs. There had been moments when I was reminded what filmmaking was all about: the commitment of a gifted crew; the exhilaration of filming a dauntless red station wagon of high-spirited teenagers crossing breathtaking country from Newfoundland to Vancouver Island; the powerful responses of other young people. But behind the scenes, the SAGE kids were having as hard a time as we were. They were exhausted, always having to be "on," and trying to get along with each other with no privacy, no rest, no time off.

Seth and I had our own difficulties. It was his first year away from home and I missed him badly. In a sense, the film made his leaving less painful, but it also presented complications in our usually smooth relationship. He was my intermediary with the group, which often caused him conflicting loyalties. He felt guilty when he couldn't "deliver" his colleagues as planned. But he also had to protect the tour from the intrusions the film made on their grueling schedule, from stops for retakes of scenic "beauty shots" (Do you mind driving up that mountain again?), to my desire to film them doing their laundry (they refused). When I arrived on the set, he expected his Mom. What he got was the Film Director, a person he'd never met before.

Every shoot ended with Seth and me apologizing to each other for forgetting our primary relationship amidst all the logistics and pressures of the shoot, and promising the next time would be more relaxed.

But the stress of working on a no-budget film was only part of it.

Shortly before the tour, I was in a car accident that shook me badly. I was coming home late one rainy night after an editing session when someone rear-ended me. I had painful whiplash for weeks. It wasn't all that serious, but for some reason I just couldn't get over it. Driving became scary, and then riding in cars. I got panic attacks on bridges and then in basement cineplex movie theaters. Over the next year the list of symptoms grew: sleeping problems, crying spells, asthma.

I suspected that I was being poisoned by the airless offices at the film board: Sick Building Syndrome. After giving me a full physical exam, Irene Kupferszmidt called it situational depression. Rather than being scared or defensive, I was relieved to have a name for what was happening.

The diagnosis made sense. I was living in the same house with a stormy, adolescent daughter and a mother with advancing Alzheimer's disease. Studio D was dying or dead, and the film board itself was floundering. At times my filmwork against violence and war filled me with paralyzing hopelessness.

I was even questioning feminism—my firm identity for almost twenty years. Feminism's gender analysis had opened my eyes, but now that vision seemed to obscure other ways of looking at the world. Many people, women as well as men, seemed to be left out. Kathleen Shannon, executive producer at Studio D, and one of my mentors in feminism, had refused funding for *Mile Zero,* saying the resources for women's filmmaking were too scarce to support a film that was not specifically about women. My head agreed but my heart rebelled against this limitation. "Doesn't the world need everyone's best energy if we are to heal?" I asked in endless arguments inside my own head. "If violence in this society is mostly male, shouldn't we welcome the voices of positive young men?" My accustomed identity was shifting under my feet. There was nowhere left to stand.

Irene Kupferszmidt prescribed small doses of an antidepressant to break the cycle of sleeplessness. I was desperate enough to take it despite my usual resistance to medication. She also advised psychotherapy. After meeting a half-dozen counselors, I started seeing Michele Devroede, a Gestalt therapist whose quiet centeredness attracted me. I told her I wanted help to slow down, find balance, and start living in the present moment.

∾

Lying in the hospital bed, I thought of all my doubts and wondered, could this stroke be what I needed to make changes in my life? My days now consisted of swallowing exercises and the excitement of walking twenty feet with the walker. Maybe this experience was a message from my body: its way of telling me something important. I remember joking that *my* body had to shout *really* loud to get my attention.

Seth suggested that if I couldn't make films, I could become like the *Speaking Our Peace* women. I think he meant that I could speak and work directly for the causes I believed in, and not hide behind the camera. I didn't need a label or job, I could be a full-time, frontline activist, unmediated by institutions. The women in my film had become role models for Seth, and now he was offering them back to me.

Seth: I think my role was to be positive. I always assumed that whatever had happened was over and now you would get better. I would hang out in your room discussing the parallels between the peace movement and your recovery. We agreed that the greatest challenge was overcoming the sense of "What difference can I make? It's out of my hands." Approaching the problem with the right spirit seemed to be as important as finding solutions. In both cases no one could know where things would end up; just moving in the right direction had to be good enough.

Seth kept saying how much worse it could have been: my mind was not affected. Although my speech was slurred, I was able to communicate. And I would surely get my strength and balance back with enough perseverance and hard work. Maybe I'd have to go to a rehab center for a few weeks, or maybe I could do it all at home.

Michael: By that time, we weren't really scared any more. You were still weak, but you were able to get up and your speech had improved. I thought you would be out in another couple of weeks and then you'd have to go to rehabilitation, probably as an outpatient, probably for a couple of months. And you were saying, "A couple of months? I don't have time for this!"

I was getting itchy about how little you were up with the walker. I felt that strengthening your arms and trunk would be useful. So I asked the physiotherapist to hook up a trapeze-like arrangement over your bed. I thought at the very least it would be useful to help you shift yourself in bed. I encouraged you to do some chin-up type things just to have some exercise. Nobody questioned it.

August 19, 1987 was our twentieth wedding anniversary. Our tradition would have been to go out for a nice dinner with Seth and Naomi. Michael and I never thought of anniversaries as *à deux*. In fact, we joked in our family that we might never have been married without Seth, so celebrating with the kids seemed only right.

~

When I was a teenager, my girlfriends and I agreed that being pregnant was the worst reason for getting married. But the road to hell is paved with such correct ideas.

When I was twenty-six and working in New York City, I was invited on a camping trip to the Virgin Islands with my friends, Bob and Sandy Erickson and their two-year-old Andrew. They had already invited some mutual friends, plus this guy Michael, whom they knew from medical school, and his little girl.

"That sounds OK, but you'd better tell him that you've also invited me," I said. They checked with him and he said "I don't want some single woman along; I don't want a two-week blind date!"

"Well, fine," I said, "I'll go somewhere else. It's no big deal to me." Bob and Sandy were always trying to fix me up with doctors, and I always refused because doctors were too boring. So I didn't have any big plans for this guy.

But Bob said, "No, damn it, I'm not going to let Michael Klein tell me who goes on my holiday!"

Bob eventually worked it out that we'd both come (but not as a date!) Meanwhile Sandy told me a bit about Michael: he was divorced, political, and had a three-year-old daughter who lived with her mother on the West Coast.

At the airport waiting for the plane to Puerto Rico, I finally met Michael. I gasped. No one had told me he was beautiful (or that his eyes matched the green of his Ethiopian Airways bag).

So there we were on the "vomit comet," the midnight plane to Puerto Rico, full of people going on holiday with little children on their laps (vomiting). His daughter Misha waltzed up to me and flung herself on my lap, grasping a book by P.D. Eastman called *Are You My Mother?* She sat with me all the way to St. Thomas, but Michael made a point of ignoring me. A plane ride to Puerto Rico, another plane to St. Thomas, a ferry to St. Johns, a stop for food at the camp store—and still not a single word.

At the camp store there was a man buying hamburger, a lawyer who turned out to be from Philadelphia like me. He invited me to come to their campsite for dinner. (I didn't know he would turn out to be a famous conservative senator!) "Sure!" I said.

Setting up our camp, Michael broke his vow of silence to tell me that I shouldn't have made this date, because our group had been expecting me to be there for dinner and he had bought food for everyone. I went on my date anyway, but came back early. Our gang was sitting around the camp fire. Michael was playing harmonica. Soon, the two of us wandered off to the beach to talk about our anti-Vietnam War activities. We ended up in the sea, and later in a camp cot. I didn't know if this would turn out to be a vacation fling where we would never see each other again in the real world, and I didn't care, although this wasn't my usual behavior even in the sixties.

As it turned out, we saw each other daily back in New York. After a few months of romance, I started wondering if it was smart of me to get so involved with a recently divorced father. Half-remembered magazine articles fuelled my fears. I was on the verge of calling it off when I discovered I was pregnant. We were using a diaphragm and spermicidal jelly, a contraceptive method which is supposed to be 94 percent effective. But someone has to be in the other 6 percent.

Our immediate reaction was to try to get an abortion. But these were the bad old days when abortion was not available—even to medical interns—except in back alleys. We were given the name of some minister in the East Village who knew someone who did abortions. It was a kind of underground church-basement thing, and it felt so creepy that we couldn't go ahead with it.

These were also the bad old days of the Vietnam war, and like so many others, Michael actively opposed it. He had been refused conscientious objector status because, as a doctor, he wouldn't have to kill people. But as far as he was concerned, to be in the military keeping other men in good health so that *they* could go out and kill people was not much different. There was no way he would serve in the armed forces; he had decided that if he was drafted he would either go to jail or to Canada.

I said, "If you make the choice to go to Canada, I will marry you and go with you and have the baby." I was a little hesitant about going to Canada with a man I had almost broken up with two weeks before, but there was no way I would marry him if he was going to jail. Michael chose Canada.

⁓

I think it was Michael who dreamed up the anniversary party; he was always pushing the rules, but this time the staff didn't mind. We had staked our claim to life in my room.

> **Seth:** I remember that party. It was just the four of us. You wanted to try the ritual your friends had done on the mountain. Everyone had a hand out and a ball of yarn would be passed crisscross through all our hands. Every time someone took the yarn they would keep a corner, and they'd say the name of somebody they wanted to call into our circle. It was like a web of yarn and friends. You said your mother's name, and Dad said his parents'. I named all the women from *Speaking Our Peace.* I was on a big evangelical peace kick, just off the SAGE trip, riding the optimistic wave I had been preaching all year. You and I shared that optimism, Naomi was a total cynic and Dad was Mr. Reality. But they still got into the ritual.

I was amazed that Michael and Naomi let down their guards and participated so wholeheartedly. Afterwards, Michael gave me a delicate cross-sectional slice of amethyst-colored quartz. I couldn't believe it—my tough-minded spouse, indulging a belief in the healing power of crystals. Whether it was my belief or his he was indulging, I don't know. On one of my purple-flowered notecards, he wrote:

What a celebration! It is a celebration, wonder at survival and wonder at how good I feel about you, us, the kids in the face of such a terrible event. I know you, we will get through it—better than ever. Love is not strong enough to explain what I feel. It is that and awe and warmth. You are my friend.

That night I was giddy and wild and happy to be alive. Twenty multicolored balloons bobbed over my bed. Bernard and his partner Isabel joined us and I held court in my hospital bed, with a rubber feeding tube dangling from my nostril, and an IV tube hanging from my wrist, showing off my chin-ups on the trapeze device that Michael had found. He said I looked like a buccaneer with my eye patch.

I remember the food! Baguettes and brie from a good French pâtisserie, caviar, dark bittersweet Belgian chocolate. And champagne! Naomi had organized it all, and was delightfully pleased with her expertise. Unfortunately, eating was a purely voyeuristic activity for me. The supplement served elegantly down the nose was my only choice. But Isabel gave me a tiny sip of champagne which I managed to swallow without choking too much. We joked that it made me even more unbalanced.

After dinner, Michael projected slides onto the wall at the foot of my bed. He'd been going through our old pictures for days, late at night when he got home from the hospital. He said he wanted me to be able to hold an image in my mind of the active woman I had been, and all I had to live for. But at first the slides just made me sad. I looked so young and athletic and healthy.

CLICK: January 1967. Michael teaching me to snorkel in the Virgin Islands National Park.

CLICK: The wedding party: Only a few intimates made it to Connecticut. Michael's parents, Annie and Philip, arrived breathless, direct from Expo '67 in Montreal. I worried (needlessly) that they weren't very pleased that Michael was marrying me, because I wasn't from an intellectual or even educated family. My parents were (very) small business people, while Annie was a retired elementary school teacher, and Philip was a screen animator, blacklisted from Hollywood for his left-wing politics. In the slide they look healthy and relaxed.

Next to Annie and Philip, my own parents look miserable. My father, recently recovered from yet another heart attack, is white and drawn, a ghost of the fat and gregarious Nat of my childhood. He has endured a four-hour car trip from Philadelphia because his baby daughter is suddenly marrying a man he hardly knows. Next to my father is my brother-in-law Bill Frankl. He is not smiling. A physician himself, he is worried that I'm throwing my life away because Michael will never be able to practice medicine as a draft-dodger. Next to him, my sister Razelle, nine years older than I, looks equally solemn. Their two boys, my nephews Victor and Brian, stand uncomfortably hot in their suits. Michael's younger brother Henry is not in the picture—he's taking it.

CLICK: September 1967. Michael at Expo, with a view of Montreal behind him. We crossed the border and were welcomed to our new city in the middle of the night as draft-dodgers. We felt like part of the celebration of Canada's 100th birthday.

CLICK: May 1968. My parents hugging baby Seth. My father died on Seth's first birthday.

CLICK: July 1971. Naomi naked in the wading pool with Seth as Underpants Man pouring water on her.

CLICK: Winter 1974. Naomi and I riding camels on a shell beach in Israel; (CLICK) swimming in the Red Sea; (CLICK) Michael drinking Maccabi beer in a field of poppies near the Lebanese border, the hulking silhouettes of tanks behind him; (CLICK) Seth talking to an Israeli soldier at a machine-gun emplacement.

CLICK: August 1977. Michael and I barging on the Canal du Midi in the south of France; (CLICK) me working locks with lockkeeper.

CLICK: 1981. Naomi with her new puppy, Lucy, in her lap.

CLICK: 1982. The New York premiere of *Not a Love Story*.

CLICK: 1987. Desiree, Alison, Max, Seth, and I goofing around at the "Mile Zero" marker bench in Victoria, B.C.

By the end, the slides had worked. I had everything to live for. I felt blessed.

◈ Interlude: Wake Up ◈

Journal: August 19, 1994

Our twenty-seventh wedding anniversary.

I came outside to do some writing and am now too steamed to concentrate. Vancouver is physically well-ramped, but that doesn't mean all the people are equally sensitive! En route to my "office," I encountered a truck parked across the curb-cut by my building, which is my only access to the sea wall. Granted it is not a designated access ramp, but there is no other route I can use. So I reached into my scooter pack for the polite version of my windshield sticker: "You are blocking my access. WAKE UP!" with the universal wheelchair graphic. (The less nice versions range from a pig driving a car that says "OINK OINK" to "Wake up ASSHOLE!"—Michael's style with computer graphics is rather less lady-like than mine.)

Along came the director of the management company for our condo. He pointed out that there was no reason for the truck driver to know it was an access route. I asked why our condo council hadn't put up a sign as I'd requested, since the curb-cut is frequently blocked, often by residents themselves or service people or moving trucks. He said he had been instructed to write a letter (the meeting was almost four weeks ago) informing me that the council doesn't want a sign. "It would ruin the aesthetic of the front walk. Besides it's not really a wheelchair ramp."

"What is it then?" I asked.

"It's for garbage disposal."

"I can see that. It is too steep to be a regulation wheelchair ramp. But the fact is, it's all we have, and there are now three people in our building who use wheelchairs on it, so I'd say that makes it a wheelchair ramp." (I hadn't eaten lunch yet; hunger gives me an edge.)

"Well, the council doesn't want to put up signs," he repeated.

"Tell me what their reasoning is, since I haven't received the letter yet."

"Well, it probably has something to do with liability."

He wanted to continue muttering but I stopped him because I was going to explode. How many times have I heard about "liability?" Last month the council decreed I couldn't park my scooter Gladys outside our unit, because it might be a fire hazard (blocking no doors in the six-and-a-half-foot wide hallway) and they would be liable. I can hear myself, my voice becoming hard and shrill. Maybe this is why some people with disabilities become bitter. But being a "good crip"—forever polite and understanding and accommodating—is making me sick.

How do you spell AUGGHH!

~

I sat on my park bench for hours, trying without success to let go of my anger and settle into writing, and remembering that other anniversary night in the hospital. When I finally gave up and came back home, I asked Michael if we had made love that night after everyone left, our usual anniversary ritual to ensure a sexy year. He replied with an atypical clarity of memory that we didn't. "How come?" I asked. "By the end of the night you were not feeling so great," he said.

STROKE TWO

❋ August 20 ❋

Michael: It was a very blurry time for me. All I know is that the day after our anniversary you were decidedly less well. You were having trouble with swallowing, transferring, sitting up, bearing your weight. You couldn't use your walker to get to the bathroom. You took a few steps and then collapsed. We joked that it was the champagne ... but I was starting to get worried. No one else was particularly concerned though.

I don't really remember that day. August 20; another hospital day, my fifteenth. Exercises. Peri-care. Maybe I felt sluggish. I remember telling Michael I was feeling worse. But how do you know whether it's serious, or a temporary setback? A bad hair day?

In the afternoon they sent an orderly with a rickety

wheelchair to take me to the gym as Iolanda had promised. I got to wear shorts and a t-shirt instead of my nightgown. The gym was windowless and dark. There were only a few other people in there, lost in their separate struggles, their voices echoing off the concrete walls. I had looked forward to it but the excruciating work made real to me how weak I had become. I was on a mat on the floor, first lying down, then sitting. Arms out. Arms back. It was like being on a little raft on the ocean of the gym floor, hopelessly rowing toward some ever-distant land, with Iolanda, my own personal cheerleader, on board.

When I went back to my room I fell into bed and stayed there for the rest of the day. The medical notes say I "complained" of cramps and nausea. I remember I played Bach's *Suites for Unaccompanied Cello* over and over.

❀ August 21 ❀

Pt doing poorly at physiotherapy—difficulty finding legs in space. No headache—no new ocular problems. R ptosis, R facial weakness, tongue to R. Speech dysfunction unchanged.

I woke weak after restless sleep. Michael came in early and stayed all day. I did my exercises up in the chair for an exhausting forty-five minutes: raise left knee, up, hold, relax, and again. Raise right knee, up, hold, relax, and again. Yes Iolanda, I'm trying, it's hard. Suck, swallow, cough. Again. The walker—proud achievement of the week before—was impossible without support.

Terre Nash: The first time I was allowed to visit you was a few days after your anniversary. You still had balloons hanging from your bed. You were tired, your speech was quite slurred but you were cheerful. You just couldn't figure out what was going on with your legs. "Look," you were saying, "I can't stand up, it's the strangest thing. And my arm just floats off—see that—I'm not lifting it; it lifts itself."

The medical team must have decided to worry. I was sent for another CT scan which showed nothing they could interpret or theorize. No new bleeding. Nothing. The neurology resident signed out for the weekend. The attending neurologist was already gone, leaving frightening instructions for what to do in case of hydrocephalus or a further bleed. By that evening I was falling over whenever I tried to sit. Falling to the right, always to the right. Michael seemed to find that significant. Me, I was too tired to wonder, drifting in and out of dreams: *something about the border, trying to cross the border.*

❋ August 22 ❋

01:30   pt slept @ short intervals talking incoherently in sleep
04:30   induced to urinate
07:00   hair shampoo—slept well afterwards
12:30   acupuncture treatment given
14:00   back to bed pt very weak

I had been working hard, I had made progress, but from the morning after our anniversary, the direction changed. I was losing ground—literally. I could no longer stand. I needed people's help to walk to the bathroom. Then I couldn't walk at all and they had to bring a commode next to my bed.

The medical notes use the words "pt discouraged" several times. I was only now recognizing that this was serious, that I wasn't necessarily going to win. I needed to cry; I knew it would be good for me. But I couldn't. When I wasn't "discouraged" I was "alert and smiling." How alert could I have been when I barely remember anything? Why would anyone be smiling? Was this all conditioned "good girl" behavior? To be cheerful and uncomplaining, to make those around me comfortable? Or was my mind somehow affected by the stroke too, in the same way my mother became more pleasant and funnier with Alzheimer's than she was before?

Physio was hell. Iolanda's cheerleader act was wearing thin as I struggled through the easiest of exercises. Don't give up. Don't give up. I couldn't handle sucking ice cubes. I could hardly swallow. I was racked by coughing spasms, bringing up disgusting, thick white phlegm. All day I coughed and choked till my throat was raw and my lungs aching. You can do it, Bonnie.

Naomi: The second stroke hit slowly, relentlessly. I remember saying to my Dad, "Dr. Afilalo said it would only get better. It can't get worse." I felt betrayed. I knew something was really wrong.

That night I skimmed the surface of sleep for hours. Every time I woke up, Michael was there holding my hand.

Or maybe it was one time that lasted all night long, or a dream. *We were in a motel near the U.S. border. Michael, Bernard, Isabel, and me. The motel felt like nowhere, like a refugee camp, a prisoner-of-war camp, with thin gauzy curtains. We couldn't cross the border. There was this question of infection. We had to pass the test, the blood test. They gave Bernard a needle. It was part of the requirement. Or was the needle infected? Was I infected? Is that how all this happened? We were behind the curtains. We had to pass the test.*

❦ August 23 ❦

24:30   unable to sleep
         neurological signs stable
         tendency to fall to R side
09:00   pt unable to stand @ all
         balance very unstable
         Mrs. Klein seems to be deteriorating ...

Michael was still there when I woke up. He helped me do my exercises. I couldn't stand. I couldn't sit. I couldn't stop choking. Something was wrong. I couldn't pee, it was too hard. The nurse put a different catheter in and left it. It felt like a piece of wire stuck up into my bladder. They sent me for another CT scan. Michael went with me. He looked at the results. He tried to find someone to discuss it with. But all the neurologists were signed out. *I couldn't cross the border.*

Michael: The CT scan was too imprecise to define what was going on. The second one had picked up some kind of bleeding, but none of the others showed anything. We needed a more accurate diagnostic tool, like an MRI, but it was the weekend and no one was there to order one. Joe Carlton had told me to be the husband and let him be the doctor, but he was still on vacation, unaware of what was going on. The ward neurologist was off studying for her specialty exams. The Chief of Neurology was gone, the covering neurologist was gone, and you were signed out to another neurologist from another hospital, who never came and didn't even know anything about you except by telephone. I would have been delighted to drop back to the role of husband if someone had been there to play the role of doctor.

Over the weekend you lost your leg function completely. You were coughing and spitting up frothy sputum and could no longer suction yourself. Up until this time your thinking had been unaffected. Now your mental functioning began to deteriorate. I called the Chief of Internal Medicine to try to mobilize some care and diagnostic skills. He promised to organize consultations for Monday afternoon.

This was the worst time I can ever remember. I stayed at the hospital around the clock, all weekend, but I finally went home at midnight on Sunday. I was emotionally and physically exhausted. I couldn't talk to you. I didn't know whether you could hear me or not. You were slipping away and you were too sick to care. You were too sick to care about anything.

I thought you were going to die. There was nothing further that could be done, there was nobody that I could talk to, surgery was never even a consideration. We didn't have a diagnosis. What were we going to operate on? People don't operate on strokes. I just went home to bed.

The only doctor on call that night was one of my first-year, family-practice interns, Mark Essak, who was cross-covering for the neurology service.

Mark Essak: It was at the beginning of my internship. I had only done a month of family medicine and then I get a call in the middle of the night to come down and cover neurology because something was going wrong with you.

I was anxious because you were the wife of the chief of my own department. My first time covering for neuro and it's the boss's wife. Not good. When I came in to talk to you, your neck was totally stiff, you couldn't even turn it to the right. Your arms were all flexed up and spastic. It was like you were folding in on yourself. It looked like something I remembered from first-year neurology: decorticate posturing.

Michael: Mark Essak called me at 2 or 3 a.m. He told me what was happening. He told me what he was doing. He had nobody else to tell. He said he was monitoring your breathing and doing blood gases, and I thanked him. He asked me if I was going to come in, and I said no. I couldn't. I just couldn't get out of bed. Mark was literally alone in the night. But I was incapable of getting out of bed.

Mark Essak: I didn't realize this was the first time Michael had gone home in days. I didn't want to tell him that you were becoming decorticate. On one hand, he's a physician and I wanted his advice. But on the other, he's the husband of the patient. So I tried to be delicate, but also tell him the signs. Essentially he said "You're doing good. If anything gets worse, call the ward neurologist at home." I did your blood gases and then I called the ward neurologist just in case. She said I was doing fine. So I just kept on.

He kept asking me questions and pulling me back. He was a sweet scared young man and I tried to help. *There was a gas or a drug that I had to take. I needed the gas to breathe, but what I was breathing was poisoning me. There was a countdown, like the creeper at the beginning of a film: 10, 9, 8; and a voice-over saying if I breathed the gases from midnight to 8 a.m., I'd be able to stop and go to sleep. But what I had to breathe was something that was killing me. I remember saying, "They promised that it would end at 8 a.m. But they didn't keep their promise. They lied."* And then Michael said, "It's OK. You're OK. It's just a nightmare."

❧ August 24 ❧

```
24:00    Neuro signs deteriorated
         L arm decorticate, grip weak R moderate
         L leg weak, R no movement
         reflexes absent—responds to pain only
03:00    movement in both limbs absent
         MD notified
08:30    lumbar puncture done by Dr. Danys
         seen by Dr. Melmed, seen by Dr. Frank
```

Michael: I slept for about four or five hours and then I went back in. Mark had taken care of it all. I'd had some sleep, and you hadn't died. If you had the will to not give up and die, then I would find the will to keep fighting too. I got on the phone and rounded up a few more specialists for the diagnostic conference the Chief of Internal Medicine had promised me. That was how I stayed sane—by banging on the system.

Naomi: That morning you were a lot worse than the day before, which was pretty bad. I read you a poem I had just written.

> Dear Mummy,
>> I envision your being.
>> A clear light,
>> It embraces
>> And warms me
>
>> The clarity of your light
>> Has shone through to my being
>> As a never-ending source
>> Of soothing strength
>
>> The generosity of your love
>> Is the sharing of your light,
>> Softly glowing between
>> Mother and daughter
>
>> Your love
>> And your light
>> Cradle my fright
>> As they sparkle through
>>> your pained exterior
>
>> I give to you now
>> what you have given to me,
>> Cling to it with me
>> As it gives strength to us both.

But you were too sick to really listen. You were having trouble breathing. Each breath was loud and gasping. I didn't get much of a response.

I think I sort of deluded myself. I felt that since I had poured so much emotion into the poem, you would respond, and it would make you stronger or something. But if someone's really sick, you have to realize when you're doing something for them, and when it's really for yourself.

I felt very deeply about that poem. I made people read it to me over and over. I felt a special bond with Naomi. Somehow she seemed to sense how I was feeling more accurately than anyone else, and for that reason I was more honest with her than with Michael or Seth, whom I protected. I worried about laying all that on Naomi, at seventeen, but her poem said she wanted me to tell her.

All afternoon, doctors and nurses and people I loved came and went and I was too tired to pay attention. I think Naomi was stroking my forehead. I think Michael was trying to explain something to me. It was real while it was happening and then it just drifted away. I was somewhere else, a place like a film loop that just keeps playing around and around.

Naomi: I came back for this big diagnostic conference that looked pretty useless to me. I remember coming in and there were like ten doctors, and one of them thought you had a malignant tumor, one of them thought it was a regular stroke, one of them thought it was what it actually turned out to be: a stroke from a vascular malformation, and one of them said it was multiple sclerosis.

It was spiraling out of control. I remember asking Dad, what's going to happen, is she going to die? And he said, I don't know.

Michael: They didn't have a diagnosis for days. On Monday the 24th, the Chief of Neurology returned. He gave a dismal assessment, feeling that it was a very aggressive cancer that was extending and infiltrating up and down the brain stem, knocking out the tracks and cranial nerve centers. He said you were probably going to die. And I argued with that. Maybe it was denial, but I was trying to figure out how he knew that. He said, "That's the way it's behaving." Which was possible. But I didn't believe it.

Another diagnostic possibility suggested was a very aggressive form of multiple sclerosis. So they called in an MS specialist, and he diagnosed fulminant MS. He saw the disease that he knows. Then they called in the vascular specialist. He saw severe vasculitis. It was a joke. I kept saying, "Wait a second. None of these things fit the pattern."

The only hard fact was that hemorrhage in the medulla which showed up on that early CT scan. It didn't make sense to say that there's vasculitis plus the hemorrhage, or that there's multiple sclerosis plus the hemorrhage. I kept saying, "There's one disease going on here. This is a healthy person who has had a single catastrophic event that is worsening. Why are we looking for several diagnoses?"

Cheryl Levitt: I was the Deputy Director of Herzl at the time, Michael's second-in-command. As you started to deteriorate, Michael phoned me at home and cried a couple of times. One morning I was seeing patients and he asked me to come to his office, so I came in and held him while he cried. Usually he was like the rabbi of Herzl, who everyone else came to with their problems. Now he was crying in his office.

And then he'd pull himself together and turn the hospital inside out for you. He was relentless. It's very much his way of handling things. Whenever I get fifty messages from Michael on my desk about things that need to be done right away, I know that he's out there trying to keep something together. He drives some people crazy. But in the end, he gets things done.

❊ August 25 ❊

24:00	heartrate elevated to 128-188
08:00	c/o difficulty breathing—drowsy
11:00	plasmaphoresis 2.5 L exchange
	incontinent
14:30	transferred to NICU
16:00	intubation w/ naso-tracheal tube

I was too sick for my own room. Everything was moving backwards. I was in neuro intensive care again. That day I shamelessly shit my bed. There was no way I could get the bedpan by myself. Maybe I called for help and they didn't get there in time. Maybe I didn't even think to call for help. I had a cheery visit with the orderly as he cleaned me up. Embarrassment was a distant concept. Breathing was more immediate.

I got high-dose steroids and two experimental treatments: Cytoxan, for my alleged multiple sclerosis, and plasmaphoresis, where they exchanged my old blood plasma for new and better blood plasma. And I was intubated: a naso-tracheal tube was inserted into my nose, down my windpipe and through my vocal cords, which meant I couldn't talk anymore. It's just a temporary measure, they said. Don't worry. The other end of the tube was attached to a respirator. To breathe for me.

The intubation was a precaution—necessary for the long awaited, long delayed Magnetic Resonance Imaging across town at the Montreal Neurological Institute. All I remember is a lot of initials—MRI, MNI—an alphabet soup of confusion. I know Michael was pleased that at last I was having whatever the MRI was.

Michael: MRI transforms electromagnetic signals into detailed pictures of the inside of the body. There were only two machines in all of Montreal, one French and one English, both with long waiting lists, so they don't push it except when it's seen as essential. But after everybody came back from their weekends, they finally agreed that it had to be done.

We went to the Montreal Neurological Institute by ambulance. I had to fight to be able to ride there with you. You were a little disoriented and I didn't want you to have to make the trip without someone you knew. I asked the ambulance attendant what method he would use to clear your trach, since without frequent suctioning you could drown in your own secretions. He told me he had an electric vacuum suction device. "What happens if it fails?" I asked. "It never fails," he said. Suspicious bastard that I am, and a firm believer in the many versions of Murphy's Law,

I asked to delay slightly while I ran up to the maternity suite to obtain a few De Lee oral suction traps (simple devices powered by someone sucking on one end). And of course halfway to the Neurological Institute the suction machine did fail, and I used the De Lees till we got there.

My memory is that all this took place in the middle of the night, but I doubt if it did. I had no sense of time or place. Joe had told me that the MRI was like a tunnel. In my mind, I saw it as the tunnel between the buildings of the Royal Victoria Hospital, where Seth and Naomi were born.

I was outside, then I was inside. I was waiting in a dark tunnel between two big Victorian greystones. It was like a bridge, or maybe it was a narrow corridor. Michael was there, then he wasn't there. My voice echoed after him, down the tunnel. But it couldn't have been my voice. I didn't have a voice.

ICU-type patient:
comatose, needs frequent suction.
Pt very spastic—took 1/2 hour to set up.

Gilles Leroux: The MRI machine is like a tube, ten feet long. Inside is the table of the magnet where you're lying during the examination. We transfer you onto a special stretcher, because in that magnetic environment a metal stretcher cannot go in. Even a credit card should not go in because it will be erased.

It was a premiere for us. A patient on a respirator we normally don't do, because there's too much metal and it's risky with the high magnetic field involved.

You had the breathing tube in your throat which was OK, it's just plastic, but instead of a metal respirator in there with you, we gave you oxygen from a rubber anesthetic bag.

At the beginning, Michael was a bit, well, he was a bit pushy. The atmosphere was quite tense. Maybe because we were groping, we were a bit nervous and he was nervous too.

Michael: I *was* pushy. I wasn't yelling but they could certainly tell how anxious I was. There were a million problems. They don't do people on respirators. They don't do people in comas. You weren't in a coma, but you weren't in control; you had muscle jerks and spasms. They need you to lie very still for a long time in the MRI or they can't get a clear image. They kept trying, but finally the chief technician said, "This is hopeless. We can't do this study. She's moving all over the place."

I basically begged him. I said, "We don't have a diagnosis and my wife is going to die without it, and I want to know what's going on." And he rose to the occasion. He crawled into the tube with you and held your head still.

Gilles Leroux: Your head was right in the middle of the magnet, your feet were just sticking out at the end of the tube. There was about five feet of space at the top, so I had to climb there to hold your head during the examination. Michael was down at your feet handling the respiration bag. The tunnel is so small that I was in a fetal position. We were there for about forty-five minutes to an hour. Your husband said "Tell her what you're doing. She can't communicate with you, but she understands everything." So I held your head still and talked to you.

Someone was talking about credit cards. There were no credit cards allowed in the tunnel. If somebody had a credit card they could get sucked up and turned inside out by the magnetic field. We were in the tunnel, waiting. Why? Waiting for what? Maybe for the ambulance. It was hot, suffocating. I was lying there and the man would tell me the banging was coming, and the banging would come, jolting through my body, filling the tunnel with its hugeness: BANG, BANG. It sounded like a broken boiler, a steel foundry. Maybe it was defective. A high-tech machine wouldn't be so loud and primitive. It was tearing the room apart.

Michael: The MRI technicians aren't supposed to tell you the results of the test. They don't interpret the film. Your neurologist is supposed to interpret it. But while I was waiting for the ambulance to come back, I put the films up on the viewing box. Magnetic resonance images are very clear. They aren't like x-rays, they're like sitting in the anatomy lab looking at a cut section of the brain. All of the structures are there, like in *Gray's Anatomy*.

And there it was, this enormous thing right in the medulla, filling more than half the brain stem. It was horrible.

I can remember distinctly having a whole series of different responses. First I thought, "It's just too big. It can't be that big." Then I wondered about cancer. But it didn't look like cancer. Malignant tumors are chaotic, with finger-like projections that go off in all directions. This mass was cystic in structure. So I was thinking, "It's a bad location but it's not malignant, whatever it is." And that lasted for about a half an hour while I waited for the ambulance to take us back. I kept looking at the film and after awhile I started thinking. "You know, it's discreet, it's encapsulated, somebody, somewhere, ought to be able to remove it if they could get to it and it's close to the surface, at least part of it, the upper part is close to the surface, under the cerebellum." And that held me for a while. It kept me from falling apart—the idea that some kind of a wizard somewhere could reach that damm thing.

Naomi: The night of the MRI was terrible. The house was filled with people who hadn't been to Montreal since my Bat Mitzvah. Old friends. Relatives. Sitting in the kitchen looking awful. I hated it. It felt like a hotel or sitting shiva. I thought you were going to die. I wrote you a letter in my diary:

"Dear Mummy, I am so very very scared. I don't know what to say and I don't know what to do. I love you deeply and totally and I hope and pray for you but I feel so very weak with fright. I wish so much that I had taken all the kisses and hugs that you offered to me throughout my life because now that I need to have them from you, you can't give them. Mummy, please live, you have to, you can't go now. I am still a little girl and I need you."

Seth: While Dad went for the MRI with you, Naomi and I were waiting for the results with Aunt Razelle and Uncle Bill and a bunch of other people. We'd been told that the worst scenario was a malignant tumor. That would be extremely serious and you would probably die. And then we got the call from Dad that you had a mass in a critical area that had already bled twice. Everyone was shocked. Naomi started to cry. Then we all got in the car and drove to the hospital. I held Naomi's hand the whole way. It was probably the first time I had held her hand since we were toddlers. All these questions were going through my head, "What if she dies? What am I going to do? What's going to happen to Naomi? What's going to happen to Dad?" I wasn't crying, but I was scared. I was trying hard to be steady for Naomi, but in my mind I was panicking. It was only now that I realized this might be the end.

Naomi: When we got back home Dad was really dazed. He went up to his study and came downstairs with a fat medical textbook with a diagram of the brain stem. He showed us where the mass was and explained what the brain stem is. It was like some sick sort of school in our living room. I think that was the worst night. We all felt beaten.

MRI reveals a circumscribed, solitary, intra-axial, vascular, expansive lesion—typical of a cavernous angioma. The pt's neurological condition and the location of the lesion would make a direct, open operation extremely hazardous.

There was to be no more plasmaphoresis, no more steroids, no more Cytoxan. By the next day they finally had their diagnosis, and there were no drugs to fix it. I had been born with a vascular tumor, a mass of malformed blood vessels in my brain stem. Over the years the mass had weakened and finally burst, causing the stroke.

I could hardly move my arms, and my legs were completely gone. I was long past dancing with Georgio. He said he was going to send me to the Arthur Murray Dance Academy. I remember laughing. Can you laugh with a tube through your vocal cords? I tried to laugh. Everyone else was leaking panic. I understood about the mass, in a twilight sort of way. Michael explained it over and over. He said it was like a pea in a pod. That image was all that stuck with me—a pea in a pod in my brain. He projected the MRI slide on the ceiling over my bed so I could understand. I couldn't believe how beautiful it was.

❧ August 26 ❧

Michael: The next day, back at the JGH, they were looking at your MRI films and saying that it was inoperable, that there was no way to get in there surgically without knocking out critical functions. I told them, "Look, I'm not interested in your negative prognosis. Something has to be done, soon. Because the alternative is death. And that's unacceptable."

At the same time, I was questioning whether I had contributed to the new bleed by encouraging you to exercise with that trapeze over your bed. If they had done the MRI study initially, then we would have known what we were dealing with, and I certainly wouldn't have suggested that kind of exercise. So I was angry at myself and I was angry at the system too, for not having made the diagnosis. The first, milder stroke had been a warning sign that was not heeded. Of course, the reality was that the malformation was degenerating anyhow, and if it hadn't bled then, it would have bled another time.

I don't know exactly when the family started to arrive: my sister Razelle and her husband Bill, Annie and Philip, Michael's brother Henry with his new partner Lyn Charlsen, and my college roommate, Norma Zack; everyone except my mother who was lost in Alzheimer dreams, six blocks away. They say I smiled, made small hand gestures and moved my lips in silent replies to their questions. Razelle was wearing a beautiful sweater. I remember the sweater more than I remember going off later for a tracheostomy to replace the temporary naso-tracheal tube. There was a corny doctor with a mustache who said, "I call this the diamond-necklace operation. Michael will have to buy you a big diamond necklace to hide the scar."

The patient was prepped and draped in the usual manner, and given anesthetic through her naso-tracheal tube. Through a horizontal incision a routine tracheostomy was carried out. A #8 Shiley tube was easily inserted into the trachea between the third and fourth rings. The patient tolerated this well. The tracheostomy tube was sewn into place and tied.

When I woke up they had cut a hole in the front of my neck and inserted a trach tube through my vocal chords. Which meant I still couldn't talk. Don't worry, they said. *The sweater was heavy wool, hand-knit in Bolivia, with bold, multicolored, horizontal stripes. I couldn't tell her how much I liked it.* (Later on Razelle gave it to me.)

Annie Klein: I remember how happy we felt on the day of your anniversary, when Michael called to say how much better you were. And then, I remember very vividly the next call. Michael said "You'd better come to Montreal. I'm falling apart."

I cried and cried. I cried all the way up to Canada, I think. But once I was able to cry like that, then I was able to deal with it.

When we saw you in the hospital, you were surrounded by medical support systems and you looked so weak. You were drifting in and out of consciousness. Your legs were rigid, your arms curled inward. You could only move your fingers. But your eyes welcomed us.

Henry Klein: When we finally got to Montreal, Michael grabbed me and immediately took me off to the hospital. He was in a dead panic. I think it was partly because he was afraid that you were not going to survive and he wanted me to see you, and partly because he wanted everybody who was a piece of your life to be there so that you had all of your life to cling to. It was the first time I ever felt that Michael needed me.

Michael: I was losing it. I kept thinking, "There's no choice but to operate on it. She's bled twice. If she bleeds a third time she'll die." Sitting around waiting for the next bleed to kill you was unacceptable.

❧ Interlude: Stephen Hawking ❧

Journal: June 30, 1993
Confusing feelings.

I can pass. I look like everyone else except I'm on top of my sporty paisley scooter, Gladys. I look perfectly "normal." I don't drool, twitch or jerk, though I used to. I thought I'd finally learned to accept being disabled. But "acceptance" is not a one-time event, it's an ongoing process.

I met Stephen Hawking yesterday and I was scared to death. Not because he's a brilliant physicist and I could hardly understand his book, A B*rief* H*istory of* T*ime*. But because he's so severely disabled.

Hawking triggers my fear of being out of control, helpless and dependent. You'd think I'd be better at this after six years. But he reawakens the horrific memories I hold just under the surface of my skin, of when I was totally paralyzed and could do nothing but blink my eyes.

I can't imagine life without movement again. Each step was so hard to get back, I celebrated every one. I find such joy today in sailing, swimming, dancing, making love. So I understand why I was scared of Stephen Hawking. But I also felt compelled to meet him when he came to Vancouver because I wanted to learn what he has to say about disability. Thirty years ago he was diagnosed with Amyotrophic Lateral Sclerosis—ALS—and was given three years to live. He can't speak, move or feed himself. He needs round-the-clock personal assistance. He has just enough movement in his fingers to steer his electric wheelchair, and to operate a special computer attached to a voice simulator.

This unlikely man has become a hero in our culture, both in spite and because of his disability. What a strange twist on the notion of hero. Typically, heroes are large and strong, perfectly proportioned. Hawking's body is fragile and withered. There's irony in his name: he's not a hawk, he's a wounded bird.

In the afternoon before his public lecture, Hawking spoke to a group of young science students with disabilities. There was a small press reception afterwards, where Hawking was to answer questions from the media. I was there for my CBC radio series, "Bonnie and Gladys," the only visibly disabled journalist in the room.

Hawking asked his nurse for tea. She poured it into his open mouth like a mother bird feeding her chick. More than half of it streamed down a large plastic bib. It was hard for me to watch. It made me recall when I couldn't swallow and Michael fed me. But I was moved by Hawking's lack of embarrassment at the mess he was making. He kept talking as if nothing unusual were going on, and enjoyed being the center of attention.

He spoke by using his slight finger movement to select a word from a dictionary on the top half of his computer screen. The bottom half showed the sentence he was forming. He clicked the completed message to an electronic voice simulator that speaks without human inflection, and—Hawking joked— with an American accent. A whole new etiquette has to be invented around this laborious method of communication: he told us to talk among ourselves until he had prepared his answer.

When asked if he follows neurological research about ALS, he said, "I tend to avoid following it too closely because I don't want to be disappointed. I would like to hear when they have a treatment, but I will concentrate on other things until then."

That is what I have learned to do, too—with lots of help— to stop looking for a cure and get on with living. But it's easier for me—I don't have a degenerative disease like Stephen Hawking, or like Sue Rodriguez, another person with ALS, who took her demand for physician-assisted suicide all the way to the

Supreme Court of Canada. Denied permission, she received it anyway. I was glad when someone else asked the inevitable question about assisted suicide.

"I will answer," the robotic voice said. "People should have the right to die if they want to. It is one of the few rights the severely ill have left. But I cannot imagine I would ever use that right myself. That would be giving in and I don't think one should do that."

Hawking became severely depressed after he was diagnosed—suicidal. When he met the woman he later married, he says he then had something to live for. That "something" doesn't have to be a lover or family, though it often is, and was for me. On the few occasions when I had suicidal thoughts, I dismissed them because of Michael and the children, our friends and family, all of whom were pulling for me. The few people I have met who gave up, either literally or spiritually, perceived themselves to be alone in the world. Interesting that it was love and not science that Hawking chose to live for.

The issue is self-determination. No one can predict how they would respond in a situation of grave illness, and so we can't judge whether someone else's life is worth living. Assisted suicide is sometimes confused with euthanasia, when someone else—often a parent or child—determines that another person should die. However well-meaning, that decision is often based on ignorance and lack of adequate societal support to care for the person and assist the caregivers.

Even self-determination is not always simple. It's not easy to distinguish between an intense but passing anguish, a conditioned fear of disability, and a considered life decision. If anyone had asked me before my strokes if I could survive so severe an illness and the resulting disability, I would surely have said no, I would prefer to die—a "choice" that now seems almost laughable.

Few would ask if Steven Hawking's life is worth living. Apart from his scientific achievements, he is more full of life than many of us: he knows how to have a good time. I saw him playing poker with Data on "Star Trek." He hasn't lost the edge of excitement about living that comes with closeness to death. Hawking contradicts my great fear of dependence. While not physically independent, he is in control of how he lives.

We folks with disabilities sometimes cynically call a person like Hawking a "supercrip." Most of our images of disability come from myth and media and are stereotyped and extreme: pitiful victim at one end, supercrip at the other. We need many more models to choose from. Most people whose disabilities are as severe as Hawking's live in poverty; many are locked away in institutions—out of sight, out of mind—leaving the rest of us with the ignorant assumption that a disabled life is not worth living, that it is, by definition, tragic.

The metaphor of flying is common in literature and poetry written by people who can't walk; to transcend gravity is the fantasy, the dream. It's what I feel when I sail or swim or drive Gladys in high gear. I love the idea of the spirit soaring, transcending the limitations of the body. Hawking does just that; his passion for life refuses to surrender to his body's paralysis.

The image of Hawking and his irrepressible grin stays with me. I wouldn't have chosen to have a stroke and live the rest of my life as I am now, but it's what I've been dealt and I'm pleased with myself for making the best of it. While I don't want to idealize bad luck, we are more than our bodies, and there's more than one way to fly.

❧ August 27 ❧

Neurostatus: Pt trying to communicate by moving lips showing what she wants with R hand.

09:50   Mrs. Klein was provided with a magnetic letter board to enable her to communicate.

15:00   Pt seems to be complaining of pain/trach site.

18:00   TF I can concentrated liquid nutritional supplement tolerated.

Michael: The MRI images moved on up the line to the Chief of Neurosurgery. He was the first person to hold out some hope. He said it might be operable, but not by him. He said we needed somebody who had experience in this particular surgery. And very few people have any experience, because usually patients die a respiratory death before they ever get to hospital. If the patient does last long enough to get into the operating room, they can die from the surgery. It's a really bad place to cut: low on the brain stem. In the brain itself, there's room to move, relatively speaking. But in the brain stem all the structures are tightly packed together. The tracks for sensation and movement, for blood pressure, heart beat, breathing and sleep cycles are interlacing, interconnecting and crossing over. So we had to find the right surgeon. Soon.

Seth: Naomi and I weren't allowed into the intensive care unit. We could only get in when Dad was there; he could get around the rules.

You couldn't talk and a lot of the time you were sort of asleep. So when I was there I would just sit by your bed and listen to the respirator. The respirator was weird because it didn't have a regular in-out breathing pattern. It had a few short sounds and then a long sound, then every once in a while there'd be a really long pause. And right towards the end of the pause, I'd panic that it had stopped.

I didn't know I was paralyzed. I remember being surprised every time Michael told me I couldn't walk. It was shocking to hear the word quadriplegic—that was a word about other people surely, not me. When I heard things like this, I thought of them as temporary. They would go away as quickly as they'd come. It's as if the paralysis did not penetrate my inner being. I was blissfully stupid.

Michael: You seemed to understand when I talked to you. At a certain point you were able to do things like thumbs up, thumbs down, for yes and no. Or you would use the letter board to spell out words. You couldn't do more than the first few letters but I could usually guess the word from that. When you lost that ability, you would communicate by blinking your eyes.

Adrianne Sklar: I was the contact person for the synagogue. I arranged for people to take turns visiting you, so you wouldn't be overwhelmed. Michael was there all the time but he also wanted us to be there, to remind you of the things you loved in life. You were lying in a fetal position. All you could do was blink. It was terrifying that you were alert and could understand everything, but I had to act as if I wasn't terrified and try to speak semi-normally.

Yvonne Steinert: I was working as a psychologist at Herzl. You and I had been good friends for years, and I would come and sit with you sometimes. I wasn't sure whether you even knew that I was there. You weren't responding. I remember drawing parallels in my head between you and my infant daughter. Here was this baby, who couldn't communicate what she was crying about. And there you were. I had to try my best to figure out what you were thinking.

Henry Klein: Sometimes it was just obvious, like you would be choking, and pointing to the letter board or the cardboard word chart for the suction thing. Or you made a gesture towards your mouth and it almost always indicated that your mouth was dry and we should give you ice chips. One time Michael got carried away and gave you a popsicle, and it came gurgling out of your trach tube. We had to clean you up and put the suction tube down to kind of vacuum out your lungs. But it was worth it for the expression on your face when you gummed on that popsicle.

You didn't have time for bull. Things were basic: scratch my behind, give me a massage, give me some ice, get this jerk out of my space. You didn't have time for any of the niceties. It was very direct and primitive and healthy.

❀ August 28 ❀

08:30   pt alert, smiling, moving eyes
14:30   listening to music w/ husband
21:40   complained of discomfort from trach by non-verbal
        gesture from face. 2 Empracet given via Dobhoff

Which memories are mine and which are Michael's? Which have I reconstructed from nightmares and medical notes? I steal memories, invent events to fill in those blank weeks.

∼

I couldn't eat. I couldn't stand, walk, run, dance, sit or speak: "locked-in," they call it. I couldn't roll over in bed—an orderly turned me every three hours to relieve the pressure of lying in one position. I couldn't read. I couldn't turn my radio on. I couldn't pee without a tube stuck up me. I shit in a pan that an orderly put under me, or I shit my bed. I couldn't unbend my elbow. I couldn't call for help. I couldn't scratch my nose. I couldn't laugh. I couldn't breathe.

Irene Kupferszmidt: You were confined. You were imprisoned in sickness. When you tried to speak there was no sound. I was your doctor and your friend but I couldn't follow your lips. Michael understood you—I don't know how. He just looked at you and he knew what you wanted to say. He would ask, "Is this it?" and you would blink yes or no.

Your kids were with you all the time. They were so good. And they were so angry: that anger of young people. They don't always talk about the things that are the most important. They don't want to water it down with words. Sometimes with one glance of their eye you have much more than ten sentences. You were the motor of that family. Suddenly they were fragments without the motor.

I remember Naomi's expressions and the way she looked at you. She couldn't take your suffering. Often she was so angry she ran out of the room. She was angry at God, at whatever, not about stupid things.

Naomi: I was scared. Every day when I came to see you, I was afraid of what might have happened overnight. Every time I got to the hallway outside the ICU, I would wonder if you were still there.

People kept saying Daddy was too positive. But things were good in a weird way. He and I were getting along and we were getting so much support from friends and family that we all felt very loved. Dad's friends from Herzl would leave food in our milkbox—spaghetti sauce, potato leek soup, chocolate cake—and there was a parade of people at our house: grandparents, aunts, uncles, cousins, friends.

Seth: I decided my role would be to keep the house stable, playing host to this never-ending stream of people who were at our house. I could always chauffeur folks around, even though I couldn't do anything to make you well. It was very comforting to feel that your friends were so committed to being there. That wasn't true with most of my friends. They hadn't had experience with major life illnesses and tragedies, so it made them uncomfortable, and they steered clear.

Those days there were no days, just a slow torrent of minute after minute: blood pressure, catheter, rest, catheter, blood pressure, rest. Sleep was a shallow nap between one person checking my IV and another person checking my blood gases. Silence was the constantly competing rhythms of the life-support equipment. Night was when Michael went home to sleep.

Night was the nightmare loop. There were bottles of poison gas. You couldn't stop the system; that was part of the torture. It was like a deadly video game, like a closed

*system and you have no control. Push any button and the
same message keeps on flashing: bad command. But I had
the feeling that there was a way out. Maybe somebody
brighter than me could break the loop; probably Margaret
Atwood could figure it out. There was a countdown. I had
no one to tell. The nurses didn't know how to listen to me.
I can't remember how long it went on for.*

What I remember is hearing my sister Razelle cry. She
was sitting by my bed and there was the sound of sobbing.
It tore me apart. It was like she was coming to my funeral,
mourning me before I was dead. Her fear was scaring me. I
clutched at Michael's sleeve. He took her out of the room.

Seth: I didn't cry at first. Neither did you for a long time.
Dad did. I remember once we were going home from the
hospital and he asked me to drive, which was unusual. So
we were driving along and he started to cry in the car. I'd
seen him cry before, but this was different, an uncontrollable sort of cry. It was really disturbing. When he was with
you, he would be really up. He had so much more energy
than anyone else. He knew exactly what to say to keep everyone going. And then when he would leave, when he
would go home or to his office, then he'd suddenly sink. So
I felt that what I had to worry about was him and the hard
time he was having. And he would take care of all the rest.

When I finally cried, it was in Dad's office at the JGH.
Aunt Razelle was with me and maybe Dad. Then Rabbi
Aigen walked into the room. He didn't even say anything. I
just walked into his arms and started to cry.

Neurosurgery note:

August 28: There is a favorable experience reported in neurosurgical literature of evacuation of both brain-stem hematomas and neoplasm via a suboccipital approach. Will follow up.

❊ August 29 ❊

06:00   suctioned several times for s/a of whitish yellowish
        secretions from trach
10:45   pt alert, smiling
        will put out tongue, squeeze w/ both hands
16:00   pt turned and positioned
19:00   pt turned and positioned
22:00   pt turned and positioned

One day. The next day. The next day. Turn and position. Trach care. I remember always being asked to squeeze people's hands. It was one of the things I could do. Grip my hand, they'd say; squeeze my thumb, wiggle your toe. They'd stick pins in me and ask me if it hurt. It didn't.

They swabbed my tongue with glycerin. It was too soft, soft on soft, how could it remove anything? I don't remember the taste. They put moisturizing jelly on my lips—thick, gunky, greasy, petroleum taste. Where was my apricot lip balm? Henry brushed my teeth. He was thorough and gentle; it was much better than the glycerin swabs. The nurse was always cleaning the trach tube. It took hours. Or maybe it took five minutes. I would want her to be turning me, and she'd be cleaning the trach. *There was something about a smell. A concentration camp smell. There was a man. He was bald and old. I said, "You're a Nazi torturer" and he said, "Yes. You got it." There was no subterfuge.*

Suzi Scott: Your trach was infected with a bacteria called pseudomonas. It has a very distinctive powerful smell. All nurses know that smell. Your trach had to be cleaned once or twice every shift. It took a long time. Pseudomonas is very contagious, very easily spread from one patient to another.

Annie and Phil read to me from the book I had been reading in Vermont. Before the hospital. Maybe it was to connect me with my old self. Everyone was worried about my old self. The book was boring, even the first time around. But it helped me sleep. When they reached the part where I had left off, I tried to tell them with the letter board. When they finally figured it out, they were very excited. It proved I was listening. It proved I could understand. It proved my old self was still there inside.

Michael didn't require proof. Every day he would sit by my bed and explain the deeper complexities of my medical condition, while I smiled and choked and the other doctors looked away, embarrassed. I remember when he started talking about the possibility of surgery. He kept talking about London, about a guy in London.

Michael: The neurosurgeons were consulting and searching the literature for some sign of success with a low brain-stem lesion. We were all searching. Your friend Norma was close friends with a neurologist at Tufts, who had a special interest in stroke. And I had a friend from Stanford, who was now a neurology professor. So we said, "OK, let's send them the MRI films. Let's send the films to every neurologist we know." We sent them overnight delivery to UCLA, Berkeley, New York, Boston. And all these neurologists called us back. And they all said "London, Ontario."

A neurosurgeon in London, Ontario had performed successful, low brain-stem surgery, just a little higher up than your lesion. Nobody had ever done surgery that low, but this guy Peerless in London had come close.

❧ August 30 ❧

15:10   pt suctioned around 15 times today for s/a secretions
color white to yellow
rubber on trach changed
17:35   respiration 26-28/min.
pt coughing constantly—Intern called
21:45   turned and positioned
family visited

Dorothy Hénaut: On August 30, 1987, my journal says: "I saw Bonnie in the ICU today with Michael. She looked beautiful but a little bit lost. Her thoughts have lost their route to her tongue. She was bright and smiling and then frustrated. My orange flowers were up on the wall. I felt so helpless.

I did a ritual that day, walking all around the outside of the hospital, planting symbolic guardians at the four corners and saying "Stay with her, protect her, no matter where she goes."

Michael: It wasn't reassuring, it was ignorant. At a certain point, I had absolutely no idea if you were going to be able to do anything again. I was terrified. And then somebody would tell me not to worry.

Dorothy Hénaut: Part of me was absolutely realistic, but I couldn't stay with that part because I wanted to put my energy into the healing. I was keeping a vision of what was possible. I figured everybody else was being realistic as shit and the vacuum that needed to be filled was the positive possibility.

Naomi: Dorothy drove me crazy. But there was one thing that I did too. I was sitting next to your bed in the ICU. You were having trouble breathing, and I wasn't getting much response from you. I was looking at all the cards up on the wall—a wallpaper of get-well wishes. I was holding your hand and trying to concentrate my love and all the love that had gone into those cards, and trying to sort of channel it into your brain so that you could heal. I was concentrating very hard on it. But it didn't work. You didn't get any better.

Naomi and Michael's needs weren't always the same as mine. It was important to me that certain people never doubted. Even if it was off the wall, they had faith. There's a difference between that kind of faith and not being able to face your fears.

On one level, people were praying for themselves. It was because they felt helpless that they needed to perform rituals or say prayers in church or synagogue. It gave them something to do, just like twiddling the respirator gave

Michael something to do.

But it also helped me. I soaked in the energy from people's dreams and rituals. I experienced this energy in the same way I experienced the medical care. It was another modality—and I needed them all. I don't believe any less in the things you can't see. Why deprive ourselves of miracles? Even if all it did was make me feel positive and hopeful about my chances for recovery, it was important. You need to hear that there is hope.

Michael: As a completely non-religious person, I can't dismiss things like prayer melting tumors. I've seen it...people whom I know are going to die come back a year later alive and well. It happens, and I just have to accept it—not in religious terms, but as sort of a humbling experience that basically says we don't understand everything. I never say to a patient that there's no hope. Because it doesn't help and it also isn't true.

❈ August 31 ❈

Neurosurgery: Will request opinion of Dr. Peerless re: pros and cons of surgical decompression in highly experienced hands.

Seth: That was the worst time, those last few days. We thought you might die. Dad made a slide of your malformation and we all worked at visualizing the different blood cells eating it away and clearing up the clots.

It was hard to keep talking to you with no response. Dad was the best at it. He didn't say stupid things. I couldn't stay in the room with you for very long. There was this horrible smell from your trach infection. Your arms and legs were either pulled in tight or bent at weird angles. Your muscles were so spastic that your fingers were sticking out in all directions. It was really hard for me, that spasticity.

Meanwhile, I was supposed to leave for university in Toronto in just a few days. I remember asking my cousin Brian if he went on to school after his brother Victor died. And he said he did, he went right back and that was a mistake for him. It never gave him a chance to deal with certain things.

I was torn. I felt very guilty. I went to see a psychologist friend of the family. She told me I had to decide what I wanted to do, for *me*. And I realized I wanted to go to school. If I had stayed, I would have been angry.

So after I had sort of made up my mind, I went to your room to ask you. You were not able to speak, but you had that letter board.

Michael: You indicated that you were worried about Seth. I asked if you were worried because Seth was going to Toronto. And you said no. You signaled that it was the opposite—you were worried that he wouldn't go.

I was dying. That's why everybody came. To say goodbye. Michael Dworkind from Herzl came with his wife, Lesley Levy. They were my friends and they worked with dying people. They brought New Age meditation tapes and Kahlil Gibran. I can hear Lesley's voice telling me to "soften." I wasn't sure what she meant, but it helped to counter the demons and the pain. They knew how to be with me, what I needed. They had experience with death; they were ready to help me die calmly and peaceably. They were not scared.

I wasn't afraid of dying. I was sad but had no regrets, no would-have-dones or should-have-dones. I was greatly loved and had made a difference to some people's lives. It was enough.

～

Joe Carlton sat on my bed after evening rounds, just like before. He was tired and sad. I tried to tell him about the video game and the poison gas, but he couldn't understand me.

Joe Carlton: When I came back from vacation, you were completely paralyzed. It was a shock. I couldn't help but feel a certain sense of guilt and responsibility, as if I should have known. But I didn't feel blame coming from anyone in your family.

I kept going over and over all the previous decisions and assumptions, trying to make them come out differently. I had assumed we had some time. There hadn't seemed to be a reason to push for the MRI. You were stable. I certainly hadn't been thinking surgery. Brain-stem surgery is just not worth it unless it's clear that function is threatened or the thing is growing. I hadn't anticipated it was going to rebleed so soon, so badly.

Michael: In the end, it was good people making bad decisions, and the system let us down. I do blame the system. If it can happen to us, it can happen to anyone.

In modern medicine we're always blundering along, making both good and bad decisions. MRI had only been around for five years or so. What would we have done in your case before MRIs were invented? Nothing. What are you going to do, cut into the brain stem on the basis of a slightly swollen thing on a CT scan? And CT scans are only ten years old. What about before that? If the lesion had bled out when you were twenty—which is more typical of these congenital malformations—you would have died.

We both use and misuse the technology. We're just screwing around trying to figure out what's going on. It's more or less enlightened screwing around; sometimes it works.

Seth: There was something incredibly naive about my thinking that all you needed was the right attitude. I took for granted the financial and cultural advantages that let Dad call neurologists across the continent and mobilize the best possible treatment for you. When I look back, I think that if Dad wasn't a doctor, then despite all your strength and optimism, you probably would have died.

❊ August 31 ❊

1) London Ontario neuroradiologist thinks:

   the quality of the MRI films is sub-optimal

   recommends repeat studies or transfer to London for

   investigation.

2) Dr. Peerless thinks a small arteriovenus malformation in this area might be approached surgically.

❊ September 1 ❊

Michael told me I had to decide something important. There was a tangle of blood vessels. The man in London was the one person who could try to get it out. He had been practicing this operation on dogs or something. He was ready. He was a surgeon who was waiting for the right patient.

But it was risky. I could die. Michael thought we should take the risk, but it was my decision. I didn't hesitate. I tried to cross my fingers, but I couldn't. I tried to put my palms together in a gesture of prayer, but that was impossible. I think I finally managed a thumbs up. It meant, yes, we have to take the chance.

Naomi: In a way, the best night was the night before we went to London. It was euphoric. It was me and Dad and Seth and Henry. Just close family. It was about 2 a.m. and we were suddenly starving but the only place open was an all night grocery store. Henry and Seth and I drove there and we bought every junk food imaginable, the stuff we weren't allowed to eat as kids: chips and cookies, full of additives and chemicals. Dad walked into the room and said, "What is this dreck?" Then he grabbed the chips and ate the whole bag.

So there we were having an impromptu middle-of-the-night kitchen party. After all of the fumbling diagnoses, suddenly a decision had been made.

Lyn Charlsen: The last night I was there, I had a dream. I came by the hospital and told it to you before I left. There was a shower of gold, kind of like rain, and somebody told me it was you. And in the dream I thought, "Well, anybody who is manifesting in a shower of gold is going to be OK." The alchemists used to try to turn bad stuff into gold and it seemed to me like this stroke was pretty bad stuff. And it was going to be turned into gold. I remember you smiled.

❀ September 2 ❀

Terre Nash: I came over to the hospital just before you were flown out. I remember it very clearly. We were all hysterical, including you. We were making stupid jokes with Skip Peerless' name. "How could anyone named Skip perform brain surgery?" Seth was calling him Skippy and Naomi was calling him Mr. Peanut Butter and Michael was calling him the Cowboy Surgeon and you were making signs with your one finger that was all you could move. We started the Montreal Chapter of the Skip Peerless Fan Club.

Razelle: We kept thinking of that cult film, *Buckeroo Bonzai*. The hero is a rock musician, race-car driver, particle physicist and neurosurgeon. And that was Peerless. He was the fantasy hero rescuing the maiden.

Naomi: We made up songs about him. "Skippy Peanut Butter, he's good enough for me." We were delirious and fixated. "Do you think that's his real name? No one's real name is Skip." And *Peerless?* What more is there to say? It was so perfectly waspy. "I bet he plays golf," Seth said.

How could anything go wrong?

Terre Nash: And then you were leaving and Naomi was holding your hand and crying and saying goodbye. You knew what was happening. The life behind your eyes was the same life. It was like you were trying to communicate everything you were feeling through your eyes. Everybody was taking turns holding your hand. You looked at Michael at one point and your eyes were desperate. I didn't know if it was the last time I would see you or not.

Sidonie Kerr: Terre told me you were going away for surgery. I didn't know what would happen. I just kept working. Apart from anything else, I wanted *Mile Zero* to be a good film. It was *your* film, maybe your last film, and it had to be strong. I felt like a guardian or something.

Michael: We were scheduled to go to London, 700 kilometers southwest of Montreal, shortly before the Labor Day weekend. Seth had to begin university the next week, so Henry said he'd help Seth pack and drive him to London to be with you before going on to Toronto.

Quebec had an ambulance jet with a built-in respirator, and the hospital arranged to have you transported. The provincial health care system didn't fuss about sending you to Ontario because nobody in Quebec was willing to do the surgery, and they agreed it had to be done.

We went to the airport in the ambulance, but they wouldn't let me go on the plane with you: "No room, no insurance, no family members allowed." Naomi and I had to take the damn commercial flight—first to Toronto—and then change planes for London. You got in about noon and we got in around 5 p.m. It was the first time I'd been separated from you.

Naomi: We didn't know when you were going to London until the day you left. There was no notice. And then we found out Daddy couldn't go on the ambulance jet. I said I would fly with him as soon as we could get a plane.

When we were finally on our way, Dad said, "Thank you for coming. I need you." I remember thinking: "He thinks I'm here for him. She's my mother, not just his wife." I mumbled something to that effect, but I was also happy that he appreciated me.

I can hear the drone of the jet engines. I can see the skinny doctor and the blond nurse with too much makeup. I remember thinking, isn't this interesting: there's a plane that's also an ambulance, with a doctor and a nurse and a respiratory therapist. . . . It was like being in some kind of television drama.

I can still smell the nurse's perfume. It made me choke. I didn't know what to do. We were stuck in this small space and I was choking and choking and I couldn't tell them it was the perfume. There was all this emergency technology but no one talked to me. No one told me where we were, or how long it would be, or what they were doing, or who they were, or who I was. I was something between just-a-job and a-big-pain-in-the-ass. I was a bundle of cargo.

❧ Interlude: Floating ❧

Journal, May 10, 1994

I went swimming this morning. I was alone in the pool and the sun was flooding through the skylight. I was floating face down with my snorkel and face mask, vaguely wondering how long I could stay like that. The light made never-ending, ever-changing ripples in the water. It was hypnotic. I remembered being in the hospital, floating further and further away. The snorkel brought back the sound of the respirator. This was a new re-membering, opening sudden and whole out of those blank weeks, seven long years ago. My throat was dry from the respirator and I felt heavy in my chest. Each breath was a decision. I remember thinking: Is this all there is to dying? Is this how it happens—breathing gets harder and harder until it's easier to stop?

Back then, I was so sick it would have been easy to let go, except for the voices and hands, holding me, calling me. Or maybe it was a physical thing where my body still demanded the breath it needed; or perhaps Michael and Seth and Naomi were with me, pulling me back.

Our culture is so strange. We're taught to see life and death as absolute states: either you're alive or you're dead. But when I was there, hovering between them, there was no sharp border. It was nothing like the near-death experiences I've read about. No wondrous white light, just an easy letting go.

Most of the time we pretend there is no death. And I live that way too, now that I'm seven years away from it. It makes no sense.

LONDON

❋ Surgery ❋

I just want to get this part over with. I was unconscious in London and I don't remember anything. I wasn't there, I wasn't there. I have nothing to say. All I know is what other people told me afterwards. Let them write about it.

Writing this, my chest is tight and breathless. My head hurts. My shoulders and neck are stiff. I remember this feeling. My body remembers. I was *there*.

I have a sensation of being on the stretcher. Tubes. Bottles. Oxygen. I'm trying to think if I felt pain. I can't remember what I was feeling. Fear? What do you feel when you don't have the energy to feel fear?

∼

I don't remember being transferred from the airplane to the ambulance. I have a vague memory of frustration because things were taking so long. Somehow I thought the plane would take me right to the hospital and I would land on the roof and be there, like in the movies. I had no idea where I was. Then I was there. Orderlies, doors, hallways. A different cubicle in a different ICU with different doctors and the same antiseptic smell.

Skip Peerless: When you came to us, you were trached and on a respirator. I don't think there was any movement in your legs to speak of, and just a bit of movement in one arm. Minimal. But your eyes were moving in that crazy double-vision way, and I could see the humanity of you coming through your eyes. You were what we call locked in: paralyzed but conscious.

It was a long time before Michael could get to me. It could have been an hour. It could have been eight hours. I had no anchor in time and place.

There was a countdown. It was a closed system. It was a film loop. You couldn't stop it. That was part of the torture. The film went around and around, like white noise: the breathing machine, the heartbeat machine. There was no way to break the loop.

And then Michael was there.

Michael: I was tense and angry on the plane, but the minute I got to the University Hospital I calmed right down. I couldn't believe the ICU. It was staggering. They had a nurse for every patient, and a respiratory technician for every three patients. They had extra beds! It was so different from the overcrowded facilities, marginal staffing, and chronic under-funding I was used to in Montreal. There were more than 200 unfilled nursing positions at the JGH.

Bill Frankl: Razelle and I flew to London and went to the hospital. It looked like you were basically dead. I had a very bad feeling that you might not recover. Or if you did recover, you would be severely impaired.

The medical records tell me I had a CT scan the first day, a cerebral angiogram on the second day, and an MRI on the third. This time there were no nightmares of tunnels and credit cards. An anesthetist in London named Adrian Gelb had invented a respirator with no metal parts that could go into the MRI. I remember the grinding noise, like in Montreal. Then you hear the clanging. And then there are silences. You don't know what's happening in those silences— whether it's over or it's going to start again. And then at last it's over.

Michael: After the MRI, we had a conference with Peerless. Naomi, Razelle, and Bill were there, and also my friends Mickey Brennan and Linda Spano, two family physicians. We were all staying at their house while we were in London.

Mickey Brennan: Do you remember what the success rate for this procedure was? It was dreadful. I think Peerless had done six similar operations, all of them higher in the brain stem. Only two people pulled through well; one died and the other three were left seriously disabled. This was a very, very chancy thing.

Michael: I don't remember the exact statistics, but Peerless said it was dangerous. But it was also in the midline, a millimeter below the fourth ventricle. There was a possible entry point. None of the others had been that way. That's what I paid attention to, not the numbers.

Mickey Brennan: Michael was in denial, which was fine. The normal process is to start off with denial and hang onto it as long as possible. If there were two out of six, then you were going to be one of the two. There wasn't any alternative: surgery was risky but no surgery was death.

Naomi: It's called the brain stem because everything stems from there. The way Dr. Peerless explained it is that the brain stem is the source, and if you lose something at the source, it's permanent. Some of your paralysis could be a result of swelling and bleeding pressing on the nerves, and if the pressure was removed, the paralysis could be gone also, but any nerves that were actually damaged in the stroke would not recover. And if some nerves got cut in the surgery, it could kill you. I was just numb when he said that. The reality didn't hit; I couldn't make myself think it was going to happen.

I remember Michael sitting on my bed; he drew me a diagram, and explained how Peerless was going to open my skull, elevate the cerebellum, peel away some other part, and delve into something else. I think he used the word "elegant" about the approach. I couldn't take it in. I didn't know the anatomy. I didn't know anything about how you open a skull. And it was my skull! It was me they were going to carve and peel and delve into, my body that would lie unconscious on the operating table, my brain in Michael's diagram.

But Michael needed to tell me. So I listened and smiled for him. He was so pleased to have a plan! After all those weeks of waiting and uncertainty in Montreal, someone was going to do something. It was a kind of big, desperate hope. Science can fix it.

I don't think I felt fear. I was swept along by Michael's enthusiasm and his confidence. I trusted Peerless. He didn't fit the arrogant surgeon stereotype. He was calm and quiet and very much a gentleman. And everyone kept saying, "If anyone can do it, Peerless can." There was this almost God-like faith.

∾

September 5, 1987. There was a full-page article in the Saturday *Globe and Mail* called "The Death of Documentary?" It was about the future of documentary filmmaking and included a picture of me and Kate Millett from *Not a Love Story*. Peerless posted it in the ICU. I was confused by the word "death" so close to my picture. Was it my obituary? The headline kept spinning in my head.

Do I really remember that? Did I see the article, read the headline? Or is it something Michael told me about later?

∾

Michael says he and Naomi came to the hospital early and were with me until I was wheeled into the operating room. He told me the operation would take eight hours. How could anyone mess with my brain for that long?

I have a vague memory of Peerless coming in before the surgery. There was something I wanted to ask him about the anesthesia. But I couldn't talk. Maybe I wanted to tell him not to give me too much because I was afraid I would never wake up.

I can almost remember the operating room. Or I remember the memories my imagination supplied later. For weeks afterwards I kept meeting people who said they had been at my surgery. So I "remember" that it was in a big stadium filled with doctors and nurses and technicians. Michael kept saying that this operation had never been done before and was historic. So it seems to me that there must have been seats—rows upon rows of students. And big lights and video cameras. I was lying on a stretcher in the middle of the stadium. The notes say I was in the "park-bench" position, lying on my side so that they could get to the back of my skull. They must have had me strapped in because I was unconscious and paralyzed. In my made-up memory, Peerless is very cool and calm and surgical.

Michael: You went into surgery very early in the morning. What the hell were we going to do, hang around the waiting room? We all went downtown to the market for breakfast. And then we went shopping. I bought a blazer, and Naomi picked out two ties for me, the most expensive I've ever owned, that I wore for years afterwards. She bought a long dark coat for herself, a real lint collector, which she has never worn. I also bought shoes, desert boots, or whatever they're called. They didn't fit.

Naomi: My dad hates to shop. He shops like someone who wants to get it over with and for that reason he is easy prey. We went to Ports for Men and he bought two eighty-dollar silk ties, a blue blazer, and pants. They were outrageously expensive but he didn't even notice. He was like a walking zombie as the sales clerk frantically circled him, sticking pins in the pants and sleeves. It was fun. It was a way of not thinking about what was going on.

Henry Klein: On the day they decided to operate, Seth and I were driving from Montreal to London in your station wagon. We had all of Seth's gear packed in the back, because after a few days in London, Michael was going to drive him to Toronto. He was pretty wired about your surgery, and also about going away to college for the first time. It was the long weekend and there were lots of other families on the road driving their kids off to university. You could tell; there'd be the boxes in the back, the nervous teenager in the front. Seth was checking them all out, because *of course* all the other kids had exactly the right number of boxes. He was getting himself into a frenzy thinking he had too much stuff and that everybody would think he was a geek. He was afraid he wouldn't know how to make friends. He said he didn't know how to make small talk, he only knew how to talk about nuclear war.

September 5, 1987

University Hospital Operative Note

S. J. Peerless, Division of Neurosurgery

With the patient under general endotracheal anesthesia in the park-bench position, the head secured in the Sugita frame, the back of the head was clipped, scrubbed with soap and prepped with tincture of Savlon. Through a midline incision in the skin, sub-cutaneous tissue and para-spinal musculature was reflected from occiput and arch of C1. . . .

On first inspection using the operating microscope there was little obviously abnormal except that the right side of the open medulla was clearly swollen and slightly discolored with brownish tinge. It was then apparent that this swelling extended up to the restiform body and had obliterated the markings in the region of the tuberculum cinereum and acoustic area of the open medulla.

A 3-mm incision was then made over the mass in the open medulla and at a depth of about 3 mm below the surface. Old brown hematoma was encountered and removed with fine suction. The opening was then held apart with two micro retractors and under 25 to 40 times magnification the cavity was cleared of old hematoma.

Working more deeply we came first upon a large aneurysmal dilatation of a thin-walled vessel which bled immediately when the clot over it was removed, causing what appeared to be arterial blood but not under particularly high pressure to escape into the cavity. This was controlled with bipolar coagulation, the dissection carried further to uncover a raspberry-sized mass of coiled, rather large vessels surrounded by numerous small arterial vessels. The small arterial feeding vessels were individually coagulated and cut, the large mass being shrunk down with the bipolar coagulator. The whole mass was finally removed in two pieces, staying always en-tirely within the confines of the cavity.

During the dissection on the lower pole of the mass we re-corded two episodes of marked cardiovascular change with, on the first occasion, a marked bradycardia and hypotension lasting some 15 seconds and the second occasion, periods of tachycardia and hypertension. These responses appeared to be related to ma-

nipulation of a single large arterial feeder but in that it clearly
went directly into the malformation I finally coagulated it and di-
vided it with no further changes in heart rate or blood pressure.

When I was confident that the complete hemostasis had
been affected, the wounds were thoroughly irrigated with saline
and bacitracin, the dura tightly closed with running and interrupted silk, and the para-spinal musculature closed in layers with
dexon and ethilon for the skin.

Mickey Brennan: After eight hours, the surgery was due
to be finished, and everyone went back to the hospital.
Here's this little room, filled with people waiting, getting
quieter and quieter. We knew that what was coming was
the moment of truth. And there would be absolutely no
way that anything could protect us if the news was bad.

Then in comes Peerless. I remember the broad smile
on his face.

Bill Frankl: Peerless indicated that in clipping off the malformation and then excavating the blood clot, the amount
of brain involved was not extensive. He felt that you were
going to come through. I wasn't sure if he was just trying to
make everybody feel good or if this was the truth. But there
was just something about him and the entire atmosphere
that made me more optimistic.

Mickey Brennan: There was no great "whoopee!" There
was just a kind of stunned, "Are you sure? What's going to
happen now?" And in fact at that point people started to
become more worried, more concerned about what the
degree of recovery was going to be.

∽

My head was aching. Somebody was there, talking to me. One of the nurses. I remember that feeling of disoriented awakening, that process of going in and out of anesthesia. I was in the recovery room with strange nurses. Or maybe Michael was there. I remember wanting him to tell me how it went. I think he reassured me that he had seen Peerless. Yes. That was it. He told me Peerless felt it was very successful.

I was still alive.

≈ Interlude: A Silent Stroke ≈

There was a stroke before the stroke. The year before, that terrible year of shooting *Mile Zero*, panicking while crossing bridges, taking drugs for depression. I remember walking up long flights of stairs because I was afraid of escalators. I remember the night I went to hear k.d. lang at the Spectrum. The club was crowded and smoky, the concert wildly exciting. I couldn't fall asleep that night. I started to wheeze for the first time in my life. I couldn't get enough air. I snuck out of bed and sat on the rocker by the open window. Still I wheezed. Must be all that smoke. I couldn't seem to remember how to breathe. I had to keep thinking about taking the next breath or I would die. I was careful not to fall asleep.

The next day I felt better, and the day after that, worse. I didn't know what was wrong. I talked to Michael, Irene Kupferszmidt, and later Michele Devroede. We looked for reasons and there were reasons enough: my mother, my daughter, my work, my life. Situational depression—the shoe fit.

But Skip Peerless found another reason. When he opened my skull he saw the two recent bleeds plus the remains of a previous bleed, maybe a year old. A "silent stroke" he called it, small enough to go unrecognized, large enough to make me tear off most of my clothes in a fit of car-wash claustrophobia, and wheeze with asthma that never responded to the asthma medications because it wasn't in my lungs but in my brain stem.

I don't remember when Michael told me. It must have been soon after surgery because I slowly came back to myself with this new information already in place. The "depression" of the previous year, the current strokes, were all related, all caused by a malformation with which I had been born. I felt a sense of relief: I hadn't brought it on myself. There. That's solved.

At the same time, I felt slightly disappointed. It seemed as if a random accident of birth had determined that I would have these strokes. It was as if they had nothing to do with me. But I wanted a message from them, a metaphor about how to live my life. In the end I decided the strokes had many possible levels of meaning and I could use whichever I needed.

❧ Post-Op ❧

Seth: Henry and I got to London that night, after your surgery was over, and Dad took me to see you. The ICU was very glistening and high-tech, each patient in their own glassed-in cubby with all of their machines and hardware. You were lying there, your limbs all twisted up, still completely paralyzed. Maybe I was expecting a miraculous post-surgery transformation. That's when I realized the recovery was going to take a long time. I remember being very comforted having Dad with me.

The noise of the ICU never changed: soft hissing like radio static and a kind of disembodied, sucking sound. After a while you couldn't hear it. The whole place smelled like disinfectant and rotting flesh. The rotting flesh was me, the stink of infection from my trach wound. I have no memory of the other patients. It was as if I was the only sick person in the world.

I remember the headache. Constant headache. There were tests with hordes of residents and medical students coming through and poking me with pins and asking me to move things. "Wiggle your toe." They were always asking me to wiggle my toe. I would try very hard because I wanted to please them, but I couldn't actually tell if my toe moved or not. The testers didn't tell me so I never knew if I was doing it right. "Do I pass?" I was good at fingers but they wanted toes.

Naomi: They were obsessed with your toes.

Annie Klein: When we went to visit you after your surgery, your eyes were bright and alive and you were moving your right hand, and even your left fingers a bit, which you hadn't been able to do for a long time. When I was telling all this to Mickey Brennan, he asked if you were moving your legs at all. I said no, not yet, not that we know of. And he said, "That's not good. It could mean the nerves are permanently damaged and she'll be paraplegic." I guess as a physician he was preparing me for the worst. I don't know. But when we went in the next day and your legs still hadn't moved, I started to get scared.

Michael: No two strokes are alike. The recovery depends on so many things, especially the location where the damage has occurred; sometimes a fraction of a millimeter makes all the difference. Sometimes there are multiple sites damaged.

Most strokes are hemispheric. They usually cause weakness on one side of the body, and often aphasia—the inability to access language—again depending on the severity and location of the damage.

Brain-stem strokes are relatively rare and there are few survivors. Even among brain-stem strokes, there are variations, depending on how low it is, and how close to the midline. The symptoms are not principally cognitive. They involve areas like breathing, swallowing, movement of the trunk, arms, and legs. The kind of paralysis you experienced was typical of a brain-stem injury. We had no way of knowing how much of the damage would be permanent.

Norma Zack: I remember going down to the cafeteria for coffee with Michael. As we sat down, he looked around at all the people in wheelchairs, and said that he didn't know how he would cope if you ended up like that. We sat there quietly drinking our coffee for a long time and then he said, "Well, actually, it doesn't look that bad."

The legs are not moving. That's what the doctors said. The legs. The body. How could it be *my* body, when I couldn't send messages for it to move, when I couldn't feel sensation when it was poked. It. When I touched myself, I didn't know if it was my own leg or some object in bed with me. My flesh felt to my fingers like a piece of dead meat from the butcher shop. My vulva and clitoris felt like strange accessories.

Naomi: When we weren't at the hospital, my dad was on the Brennans' phone, keeping everyone in Montreal, California, Philadelphia and New Jersey up to date. The Brennans were incredibly generous with their home and they were really good at making fun of Dad. One Friday night, Linda made this amazing Shabbat dinner including the best matzoh-ball soup I've ever had—there were tiny quail eggs in the middle of the matzoh balls. And she isn't even Jewish! She set this beautiful table in the dining room and at one place she put a pink telephone right on the plate. "OK, Michael," she said, "guess which seat is yours."

University Hospital was like a posh resort for sick people. Everything was brand new and completely high-tech; all the doctors looked like they had just stepped off a golf course and taken an exhilarating shower. The nurses were big, healthy, strong, unbelievably attractive people who all seemed to love their jobs and love each other. Bottom line: they were not burnt out, unlike at the under-staffed JGH.

The nurse with the blond hair sang to me while she made my bed. Something about a bird, "with a wing on the left and a wing on the right," complete with flapping elbows. The other good nurse was Rick. His voice was very calm. My head hurt.

The nurse Rick talked to me. "Now I'm going to brush your teeth. What flavor toothpaste today? Hmmm, mint. Do you like mint? I hope so 'cause that's all there is. Is that too hard? Blink your eyes if it's too hard. OK, now I'm going to swab it out. There. So when do you get to start eating steak?"

It's very intimate to have someone else brush your teeth. Rick knew I was alive.

Seth: A few days after your surgery, Dad drove me to Toronto. I was nervous about going to university. Looking back, I don't know how I did it, or if it was the right thing to do.

When we arrived, Dad helped me move into my new room in residence. It was a small space, and without any posters or books it looked a lot like a prison cell. We stepped into the room, then Dad sat down on the bed and started to cry. I guess it was a combination of many things: his son starting university combined with the relief of the surgery.

Michael: It was a long drive to Toronto and back. So when I got to the Brennans' around 11 p.m., I called the hospital and asked how you were doing. The nurse said your condition was not good. You were less responsive and you had fixed and dilated pupils. Fixed and dilated pupils means brain-dead. It meant some catastrophe had occurred;

there'd been another bleed. It didn't make any sense to me, in light of how I saw you when I left, but these things do happen so it was not inconceivable either. I said, "I'm coming right away," and hung up.

Mickey was upstairs, asleep. I don't think I made any noise, but the next thing I knew, he was downstairs in his pajamas, asking me what was wrong. Then he was getting dressed and we were driving like crazy to the hospital. I remember this kind of empty feeling in my stomach. The nurse was waiting for us at the door to the ICU, crying. She was a mess. She said, "I'm very sorry, I made a mistake. It was another patient; your wife is fine."

Naomi: Eventually I had to go back to Montreal for school. It was really hard to leave. I got home the night before my boyfriend left for college. I spent the evening with him and he left at about one in the morning. Then I went to the kitchen to get something to eat. It was really quiet. All of a sudden I realized that I was totally alone. Our dog Lucy was at our friends the Ushers' house, you guys were in London and Seth was at school in Toronto. It was too late at night to call anyone. I started to get spooked. I was hearing noises—like footsteps on the stairs. I went into your bedroom and locked myself in. Finally I fell asleep and the next day I went to my new school, Brébeuf, where everything was in French. I was a total mess. The only good thing was when that afternoon there was a message from Dad saying you were starting to get better.

I seemed to have moved my left big toe. They said I did. I couldn't feel it, but they were very happy. I passed the test. I could move all my fingers and one toe. I could lift my right forearm off the bed. I wore moon boots. I had a dream of shit. Or maybe it wasn't a dream. *There was an ocean of diarrhea all over my sheets and bedclothes. It was sweet shit. That's what we used to call it when I was breast-feeding. When it's your baby, it's not repulsive. It was like swimming in a warm, sweet ocean.*

The moon boots were blue styrofoam splints. The physio prescribed them to straighten my feet which were rigidly turned in. I had hand splints too, to straighten my wrists and thumbs, but I used to wiggle out of them. I guess they were uncomfortable.

The Blue Chair was another torture device I was put into at intervals throughout the day. I remember dreading that chair. Sitting in it was enormous work. There was always a big deal about how long I could stay in the Blue Chair. The nurses were so excited when they could say, "Ooh, she sat in the Blue Chair for half an hour today."

Michael: The Blue Chair was a pretty standard lounge chair with a high back for neck support since you couldn't hold the weight of your head yet. The nurses would either get a couple of orderlies to lift you into it, or they'd use the hoist which was like a derrick that winched you into the air in a kind of sling and swung you over and down into the chair. Rick couldn't be bothered with that. He'd just schlep you over in his arms.

Sitting in the chair was an exercise to help you develop trunk control. You were having a hard time just staying upright. Even when you were in bed, you had to be wedged and propped, and every two hours they would turn you. Even in the middle of the night they would wake you and turn you; otherwise you would have been bearing weight on your buttocks all the time and would have gotten bed sores, which are hard to get rid of, extremely painful and can become seriously infected.

The nurses in London had a clever way of turning me: it was like that trick you see in old movies, where they pull the tablecloth out and leave all the dishes in place. Two of them would grab the edge of the sheet and flip me like a pancake on the count of three. (There was a more complicated variation for changing the sheets.) Between turnings I would just lie there, unable to move my head to look at someone or shift my weight in any way.

Michael: I remember one time you were trying to tell us that something was hurting you. We thought you were saying it was a headache. The chief neurosurgical resident came down and did a careful examination but she couldn't figure it out. You were too uncoordinated to use the letter board. Then somebody came along with a diagram of the body, and we started pointing to different parts and asking you if that was what hurt. That's how we found out it wasn't your head. As soon as that was clear, the neurosurgical resident was no longer interested and left the rest of us to figure out what the hell was wrong. We went down the diagram with you mouthing the words: no, no, no. Until we got to the pelvic area and then you were saying: yes, no, yes, no. We were totally confused until we realized that the diagram showed only the front of the body. We turned you over and, there was a big red sore spot on your bum.

In spite of the morphine they gave me, I was often in

pain. I think I kept my eyes closed most of the time. I know I was dizzy from double vision and a condition called nystagmus where my eyeballs kept bopping around. Smell was much more vivid than vision. Certain odors caused my throat to go into spasm. I choked at the smell of cigarette smoke on people's clothes. I could tell what they had eaten for supper. Strong foods were offensive, but I loved the smell of sake.

I could lift my arms off the bed for seconds at a time, and even though my right foot was still disconnected, I could wiggle my left one like crazy. I still couldn't breathe, eat, pee, speak, sit up, or dance, but surely those would come soon. Meanwhile the nurses did practically everything for me. There was skin care, back care, mouth care, bedpans, massage, bed baths. There was constant checking of blood gases, spirometers, IVs, feeding tubes, catheters, and trach tubes. The best time was Rick's shift. He had a flat, nasal, Ontario kind of voice, but to me he sounded handsome and sexy. In the warm current of attraction, I remembered I was alive. He'd tell me about his day and what he was doing and what he was going to do next: not profound talk, just talk.

"I'm thinking of buying a windsurfer. What do you think? Last weekend I tried Steve's. You know Steve? The RT's boyfriend? Anyhow, a bunch of us went out to the lake and I was windsurfing. Man, it was amazing. Just zinging over the water. And falling. Did I mention falling? OK, OK, so I'm a klutz. But should I get one? Blink if you think I need a windsurfer. All right! I knew you'd be on my side."

I understood everything. People would talk to each other and my imagination would piece together stories from the fragments. There was an ongoing soap opera in my head: *Rick and the pregnant occupational therapist were some kind of number. Whenever they were both off duty, they were together windsurfing.* But it was all in my mind. It turned out she was married to the orthopedic resident.

Michael: You used to laugh with Rick. You didn't make the sound of laughter, but you laughed. That's why Rick liked looking after you—you were responsive.

A lot of the nurses didn't even talk to you—you couldn't talk, so you weren't worth the bother. But in fact when something was working well, I could see it in your face. You'd be shining. That was real feedback if people chose to see it, and the difference with Rick was that he saw it.

Seth: I used to talk about you to the staff every time I came in from Toronto. I felt a strong need to tell them who you were—about all your films and friends. I wanted them to know they were dealing with a real person, not just a paralyzed body.

I remember one of the nurses giving me a bed bath and saying to the respiratory therapist, "She used to be a filmmaker." As if I wasn't there, as if I couldn't hear, as if my life was over. I wanted to shake them and say, "Don't talk about me like I'm dead!" But I couldn't shout or shake anyone or even explain it to Michael on the stupid letter board. I remember my finger wobbling around, not able to reach the right letter. I remember the blur of the board in my double vision. I remember the letter board getting lost, over and over again. I don't know why they didn't have an extra one?

Skip Peerless: The letter board is considered a minor item overall.

It was my life line.

❧ Interlude: Finding Memories ❧

Journal: January 1989, Costa Rica

I asked Michael to help me find memories from that lost limbo time after surgery. Michael is more interested in watching the sunset. He is casual about memory, prefers the present. But I am always working, worrying at that hole in my life. I'm afraid of what's there, but I feel I won't heal without finding out.

"Why were those splints called moon boots?" I ask him.

"I don't know. They just were."

"Did I go somewhere for the moon boots? Some kind of theater?"

"Theater? There was no theater. Hey, look at that fishing boat out there. What do you suppose they're after?"

"What about for suctioning?" I persist. "I remember some other place, a big place they took me to for this stuff."

"No, it was all in your cubicle," Michael says. "Splints, suctioning, trach cleaning, everything."

"I don't remember," I say, but suddenly I do. I can see the

clear plastic around my bed, hear the soft shush of the respirator, choking, footsteps, voices.

"We'd suction you out constantly," Michael says. "A couple of times an hour. I used to take turns with the nurse or the respiratory technician. You would start choking and bubbling, and we'd have to disconnect you from the respirator and connect you to a self-inflating bag that would take over breathing for you. Then we would put distilled water or a saline solution down the trach tube to make you cough."

He's on a roll now, explaining the procedure, and the memories are flooding back. "It was awful," I tell him. "I would cough and sputter and they would say 'good.'"

"Coughing kept you from getting pneumonia and it also cleared the tube. Then we would suction out the trach and bring up all of the pus, mucus, and debris. It had to be done thoroughly."

"I hated it."

"Yes, because it made you choke."

I remember that all right; my body resounds with recognition. But I still want to know more.

"Do you remember being weaned off the respirator?" Michael asks. "They put you on a schedule where you spent an increasing amount of time every day practicing breathing on your own."

"Was that in the theater?" I ask.

"Forget the theater! There was no theater!"

"OK, OK, tell me," I say.

"We would unplug the respirator and hook you up to a t-tube—an accordion-like tube that attaches to the trach and provides oxygen. But it doesn't inhale and exhale for you like the respirator does. As you breathed this dial would turn and indicate if you were getting enough oxygen and whether you needed to go back on the respirator. Sometimes it was clear that you'd been off for too long and were exhausted."

"I think I remember. I couldn't breathe. And you would clean the t-tube with that horrible smelling cleaner."

"No, that was for cleaning around the trach tube. The gauze would be impregnated with all this smelly pus. It's a disgusting smell: overpowering and sickly sweet. I remember you complaining about that smell on your letter board. I think it had something to do with the panic attacks."

"I don't remember," I say.

But I do.

❧ Panic ❧

Does torture have a smell? My foot was caught. In the sheet, or maybe in my nightgown. I tried to move but couldn't. I was paralyzed. My leg was far away. I couldn't find it. It was caught in a trap. I was trying to scream. The nurse said "There, there, it's all right." But it wasn't all right. I was trying to tell her. I was trying to scream. "You're fine," she said. "It's nothing."

Michael: Almost two weeks after the operation, you started having panic attacks. Some days you'd just have two or three, but other days they'd be coming every hour. You'd be dozing and then you'd become suddenly alert and there'd be a look of total terror in your eyes. You didn't have very good control of your arms, but you would clutch at me, you would clutch at the nurse. And the nurse would say, "Calm down. It's nothing."

It was not nothing; I was choking to death. I couldn't breathe, I couldn't swallow. I was drowning. What did they know? The damn letter board was lost again. *I was in the concentration camp with a torture device on my head. It was squeezing my skull. Even morphine didn't help. There were circles and squares and something about blood gases and oxygen and numbers. I could smell the cyanide.*

The singing nurse was stroking my head. Mary. Her name was Mary. I wanted to tell her about the bald Nazi. I wanted to ask her if I was dying. I wanted her to stroke my head forever. "You're going to be OK," she said. "It will pass." Michael got a big green magic marker and made a new letter board on the back of an old file folder. The letters were messy, but it worked just as well as the lost one.

Michael: I remember you trying to tell me about the nightmares, but it was a concept that I couldn't get. All I knew was there was something terrifying. I would try to acknowledge what you were going through by saying, "Yeah, it's scary. It must be absolutely terrifying. But it will pass. It has never not passed. Just let me hold you." That was the litany. It was only marginally successful.

Rick: It was as if you were trying to tell us something, but you weren't able to. You'd get a worried look, and then you'd start getting physical symptoms—sweating, agitation, labored breathing. But there was no actual physical problem. There didn't seem to be anything we could do to keep you from going into a panic attack, but once it started, if the nurse didn't take the right approach, it would just get larger.

Michael: The phone was next to your bed so that if you got particularly anxious, the nurses could call me and put the phone to your ear and I would talk to you. You couldn't talk to me, but you could hear my voice.

I was afraid to sleep because that's when the film loop would start. But I wouldn't get well unless I slept. It went around and around. Michael was gone.

It took me a long time to get the nurse's attention, and a long time to tell her what I needed. She refused to call Michael. She told me I was being a baby, that he had to eat and sleep and play tennis, so I would have to wait until he came back. She smiled and patted my hand. "He needs some time for himself." "No," I wanted to yell, "I don't care what he needs. If he knew how desperate I am, he would want to be with me and save me."

I knew he was staying at Mickey and Linda's. I tried like hell to remember the phone number, but I couldn't even remember their last names. I couldn't look up the number, I couldn't even dial, and the gatekeepers wouldn't help me. I was trapped. I would die in the hospital while Michael was playing tennis.

Panic attacks punctuated my days, feeding off the ICU atmosphere of constant hysteria, of life and death. My skin was too thin to keep it out. There was no distinction between myself and the outside world. It jolted through my nerves, made my heart race, constricted my chest. The ICU melted into the nightmare concentration camp: constant lights, constant noise, constant routines. All day and all night. I was desperate for sleep and the rock of Michael's presence.

September 18. The nurse's notes say, "pt mouthing words: 'Help me, I'm going crazy.' Settles with comfort, or at times a firm hand." My body tenses against the memory. There was a psychiatrist, someone Michael vaguely knew, who just happened to be in London. He came to see me at Michael's request. I pulled at his white jacket, saying, "Help me." I knew he was a psychiatrist, the kind of doctor who is trained to help frightened people, the kind of doctor frightened people are trained to ask for help. He pulled away, almost ran for the elevator. I could see his terror—she's insane, she's off the wall. I'm getting out of here, fast. I'm a busy man.

Michael: You let me know that you were afraid you were crazy. I said that anybody going through what you were, had every right to be crazy. It was no big surprise and nothing to be afraid of.

I suppose I was crazy. Something was going on that I couldn't control and it was driving me mad. Although it was based on a physical reality, what I experienced and the way I acted is commonly labeled insane. I crossed the line and discovered there really is no line. The division between myself and those other people, those crazy people, was gone. They were me.

I tried to pull myself together for Michael. I desperately wanted to give him a good reception, to show I was OK. Sometimes I could do it, but more often I would fall apart. I would try to tell him what I had been going through and end up making dry soundless sobs. I was angry at him for abandoning me.

Everyone kept moving around: London, Montreal, Toronto. It was a complicated choreography of comings and goings; planes and trains and cars and cities; today, yesterday, tomorrow. I couldn't understand why everyone wasn't there all the time.

Seth: My whole first term of university was awful. It scares me now when I think how cut off I was. There were only two people who knew what was happening with you, Alison and Sheila, friends from SAGE. I resolved to tell no one else. At school, I would concentrate on my studies and try to have a social life. On the weekends, I would take the train to London and focus all my attention on you and Dad and Naomi. I guess I felt guilty for leaving, especially after the panic attacks started. I came to hate those train rides, doing my homework and trying to shift my brain from one compartment to the other.

Carol Zavitz: On the day of your first stroke, I was in Toronto, giving birth to Natty, our first child. In the weeks that followed, I was entirely absorbed with that inscrutable little being who had been part of me. I was looking for other mothers who would rejoice in the baby in the way that I needed, so I called you—a longtime friend and ace rejoicer. Naomi answered the phone and said you were sick.

I think you had just gone to London. We got in touch with Michael who suggested that Dan and I come to visit you; he was concerned that you not lose touch with the world outside intensive care.

When we got there, Michael saw us through all the gowning and washing. We knew that according to the rules, we shouldn't both go in at once, and certainly not with the germy baby, but it was clear that Michael made up his own rules for your care.

You were lying on a very high bed in the middle of a bristling nest of machines. I wouldn't have known you. You were asleep and looked flattened out, obliterated. I felt I was seeing you from far away and that you were dying. It looked impossible to get close to you through the beeping equipment, to make any kind of human contact.

Michael woke you and ushered us in closer. I held up the baby so you could see him, and all at once your face came alive with an expression of joy and wonder and welcome that made the ICU recede into irrelevance. There you were after all. Excited to see a new baby, you started to talk; you had no voice, of course, so Michael interpreted for us. You got tired very quickly; two or three times you dropped back to sleep and vanished again, but now I knew you were there, just hidden sometimes.

I didn't believe you were going to die any more. I was vividly aware that you were going to have to learn, all over again, what Natty was just starting to learn: to eat, use your hands, balance, sit, walk.

We spent some time with Michael after we left you. The total integration of physician and loving husband in him amazed me. Every part of him was activated to care for

you, and to organize the rest of the world to care for you
better than it would have dreamt of without his example.

The baby was nursing in my cubicle. They were friends,
and they were sharing their baby as if I was alive and well,
as if they wanted my blessing. It situated me back in a world
of which I was not the center. The focus was clearly on the
baby; how could it be otherwise? It was a moment of peace
between the panics. Michael and Rick decided that new-
borns should visit the ICU all the time, as a standard therapy.

∼

*The Nazi came at night. I asked him if I was going to die,
and he said yes. I couldn't get away. I was struggling, choking, dying, grabbing out for someone to help me. "Don't
leave. Please don't leave."* Only Michael could talk me
down. He would breathe with me until I fell asleep. The
literal meaning of "conspire" is to breathe together. We
were conspirators against the night terrors. He would hold
my hand and breathe deeply and steadily, till I could drift
off. Only then would he go home.

Twice a day, the doctors came on their rounds. Skip
Peerless with a small army of penguins following him. It
was like a hurricane with everyone scurrying around—"The
doctors are coming! The doctors are coming!" They would
look at my chart for five seconds and tell me I was doing
great. "Good stuff, good stuff," Peerless would say. They
were delighted with my progress. I was a success, I could
be checked off. This psychological stuff was trivial and there

were lots more patients coming in from all over the world, needing dramatic surgery. No one wanted to know how bad I felt.

Michael: Once the panic attacks began, I had to start playing doctor again. You were at the mercy of whatever nurse was on duty. If it was someone like Rick or Mary, you would be in relatively good shape. But if it was one of the punitive ones, you'd be a mess. The way they would treat you drove me crazy. "Don't be a crybaby," they'd say, "There are people who are much sicker than you in this unit." Meaning unconscious people. They were great with unconscious people. I would tell them "There is a problem. She's in pain, she's paralyzed, she can't speak and she feels terrified. You can't talk her out of it because it's real." I had to constantly reassure you that you weren't being too demanding. You didn't need to feel guilty on top of everything else.

I asked one of the nurses why she was looking after you if she really didn't want to. She responded frankly that it was not that she didn't like you but the shift rotation gave her no choice. She really wanted to work on the transplants, the livers and cardiacs as she called them. Her goal was to learn how to use the new machinery that goes along with each new procedure.

Luckily, Rick was ready to take the panics seriously. He and I agreed that we needed a case conference to develop a workable approach that could be applied consistently on every shift. He spoke to the head nurse and got permission to organize a meeting. I brought literature on panic attacks. Out of the discussion came a very clear and sensible plan—you would be looked after only by the nurses who wanted to work with you and learn about panic attacks. We outlined specific relaxation techniques that everyone would apply. It made a real difference. It didn't stop the panics, but at least people were not being cruel to you.

A year later I saw an article about something called "ICU psychosis." People who spend long periods of time in intensive care often have uncontrollable fears and hallucinations, frequently related to torture. It wasn't a new concept, either; it had been studied for years. Why would highly trained people identify your problem as "acting spoiled?"

At Michael's urging, they started me on a minor tranquilizer, Xanax, and an antidepressant, Ludiomil. In my old life, I would have been wary, resistant, but now I was willing to try anything to keep the nightmares at bay.

I yearned to be in a room full of furry puppies—wiggly little golden retrievers, like our dog Lucy when she was young. I could feel their puppy-down tickling me, their exuberant licking tongues as I rolled around laughing with them. I breathed the earthy smell of their wet fur. If I could go into that room, I would get better.

Michael: I was sitting on your bed, and asking you if I could get you something. I was reading your lips or the letter board, I don't remember which. You told me that you wanted to talk to Michael Dworkind and Lesley Levy. They had experience working in palliative care and had been very helpful after your second stroke. I called them on the phone by your bed and held the phone to your ear as they talked to you.

Lesley Levy: We'd never done anything like that before—

panic management by long-distance telephone, but Michael sounded pretty desperate. It was really hard to know what to say because we couldn't get any feedback from you. If we could have seen you, we could have read your facial expressions, but there was just silence. What we did with you was a technique we were just learning—meditations from a book by Stephen Levine. We mailed Michael photocopies that he could read to you, and a tape of us reading as well. It was our way of dealing with the fact that we couldn't just hop on the plane and see you.

Michael Dworkind: You were completely dependent on others. You were being passively handled, without being able to speak your own needs. It's a horrible situation. No wonder you were scared! But the meditations were telling you that no one can take away your mind. Your mind is a tremendous, powerful tool. Even though you're paralyzed, not able to talk, you can still do something. If you pick up an ember in your hand and hold it softly, it hardly burns you. But if you clench it, it hurts much more. So there are ways of accepting your pain. It doesn't go away, but it doesn't burn you, and you can live with it.

Michael: It used to drive me nuts to read you that stuff. I despised it, it was so banal. But in fact the meditations helped. I read them day after day, night after night. What did I care if they sounded like New Age crap? They worked.

It is a cliché to be looking towards "spirituality" on death's doorstep—the old life insurance thing that says just in case there *is* a god . . . or when all else fails, pray. I don't think that was true of me, however. I wanted wisdom, help to smooth my way through the pain and the fear and to accept my illness. I had died and come back to life, stripped to the bare essentials. No speech, no movement, no breathing. What is the Self then? Who am I, with none of the usual human accoutrements, let alone my particular labels and roles? I was de-constructed, literally. How post-modern of me! It sounds pompous now, but I wanted to live through this experience well. With meaning and grace. I never considered not struggling to survive. Too many people were in it with me to give up.

> **Michael:** I made a list of all your friends in Ontario and showed it out to you, asking who you wanted to see. You pointed to Rosalie Bertell, so I called her up. She came all the way down from Toronto and prayed by the side of your bed.

Rosalie is a biostatistician who has done brave and lonely research on the cancer-inducing effects of low-level nuclear radiation. She is also a Catholic nun. As Terre and I selected the women for *Speaking Our Peace,* we didn't realize that they all had deeply-rooted spiritual beliefs, even church affiliations. Muriel Duckworth and scientist/philosopher Ursula Franklin are Quakers; writer Margaret Laurence was a United Church goer; Marion Dewar, then mayor of Ottawa, is a practicing Catholic. While we chose not to correlate their religious beliefs with their peacemaking, I knew they were not coincidental either.

So when I needed spiritual guides, the *Speaking Our Peace* women became even more important to me. And true to form, they were all there for me, with letters, visits, phone calls.

I remember Rosalie sitting by my bedside in London. She knew how to sit with the sick. "Do you mind if I say a nun's prayer?" she asked. She waited for my answer. I was a little nervous. Was it like the last sacrament before you die?

She began by "thanking God for the clean air and sparkling water, and for the precious life of Bonnie." There was also something in the prayer about God taking me under Her wing. Rosalie slid back and forth between female and male pronouns and imagery in the most natural way. I know that's not easy to do, because we stumble through it in our synagogue. "What is Woman that thou art mindful of him?"

Much as I appreciated Rosalie's prayer, I kept thinking there must be Jewish sources of knowledge about sickness and death. I longed for the illuminating humor of Jewish spirituality. Why was I so unprepared? Where was the wisdom of my own elders? What could I do to sanctify this moment? It's strange that at a time when I couldn't remember where Montreal was, these questions were so clear inside me. I was thinking of Sholom Aleichem, the Yiddish writer whose stories are so bittersweet, and all those Hasidic stories about consulting Reb Nachman of Breslov or Reb Zusya of Anipol about the ultimate meaning of life:

> ... and Reb Zusya said: When I arrive at the gates of judgment, I will not be asked "Why weren't you more like the great Moses?" I'll be asked "Why weren't you more like Reb Zusya?"

I knew these stories existed but I couldn't remember any, and without language I had no way to explain my need.

Michael: You somehow indicated to me that you wanted me to call Rabbi Ron back in Montreal, and that I should ask him to tell you something funny. All through your phone conversation, you were kind of snorting and choking with laughter. I still don't know what he said!

⨾ Interlude: Rosh Hashanah ⨾

Journal: September 7, 1994

New Year's began not so sweetly.

Michael, Seth, and I went to Or Shalom Monday evening for Rosh Hashanah services. I was looking forward to this New Year like never before. I was keen to show off our synagogue to Seth who has just moved to Vancouver to go to graduate school after teaching up north last year. Or Shalom is a community where I am at home, where the most diverse group of Jews I know feels at home.

Services were at the same address as last year—the Talmud Torah school. Last year, my first, I had carefully checked the venue beforehand, but by now I'd learned to take access in Vancouver for granted. What a shock to see the flight of stairs leading down to the auditorium.

Michael scurried to the side and rear of the building, confident there'd be another way in. We are used to service entrances and freight elevators. No such luck. It was completely inaccessible. Ellen Frank, my friend and disability buddy, limped over on her cane, looking like death. Our eyes met. Ellen uttered three words: "no one noticed." It turned out that she had been there earlier and even *she* hadn't noticed. There was no "them" who forgot; them was us.

By then, many others had arrived. Some people rechecked the building in disbelief. There was visible pain on the faces of several members of the shul, probably the people who'd worked so hard to create these wonderful High Holiday services for us. They were horrified to see me in my scooter at the top of a flight of stairs.

And probably ashamed.

And my reaction? Hurt. Isolated. Then a rush of other feelings quickly pushed those away. I was stupid for not checking it out beforehand. After all, I hadn't been to synagogue all summer, so why should other people remember? I hadn't been able to volunteer for any of the committees; other people had been doing all the work—how could I complain when they were doing their best? Most of all, I felt guilty for making them feel guilty on Rosh Hashanah.

Then I remembered I had invited my friend Pat to join us the next day. She hadn't been to synagogue for years, since ALS put her in a wheelchair. She was thrilled to be coming. I felt horrible.

I parked Gladys unobtrusively and struggled down the stairs, using one cane and clinging to the railing. I tried to let it pass and get my spirit into the services, but my head wouldn't stop buzzing. I wasn't really part of this community; I was Other. And how would I tell Pat? I was robbed of my holy day peace.

The phone was ringing as we got home. Pat wanted to

make arrangements for the morning. "You can't come. I'm sorry, it's inaccessible." I fumbled with excuses. Pat leapt in: "They're good people. We have a year to teach them—this is good." I learned later that she wheeled down to the ocean and cried.

The day after Rosh Hashanah, I flew to the Okanagan Valley to attend a workshop of the B.C. Coalition for People with Disabilities. The others had gone by bus two days before; I had stayed for the holidays. At the end of a stimulating three days, with a sense of belonging to this community of people with disabilities, I stood up as a Jew. I told them that just as I would speak in my synagogue about "reasonable accommodation" for people with disabilities, I needed to call their attention to the fact that they continued to schedule major events on our most important holidays. Maybe they could make "reasonable accommodation" for people's religious priorities.

Afterwards, though, I was plagued by doubts. Was I too demanding? How much is too much to ask? How much should Or Shalom or the BCCPD have to give up in order to accommodate just a few people?

Why do I still feel that it's asking too much to want to be included: as a person with disabilities and as a Jew? Our rabbi spoke about stretching ourselves that extra bit when we thought we'd stretched as far as we could. I will use this Rosh Hashanah to commit myself to speaking my piece, "making a stink," as Marsha Saxton, one of my disability mentors, says, wherever and whenever I can, even at the risk of being a nag. I will invite people to be our allies, not out of guilt, but in the spirit of the Mitzvah of Tikkun Olam, rebuilding the world. Maybe literally.

~

September 1995: Update
This year's High Holiday services will take place at the wheelchair accessible gym.

❀ Leaving ❀

Anne Usher: Michael phoned me and asked if I would come visit in London. He's usually so strong and analytical and together, but this time he sounded really lonely. I think he probably hadn't been sleeping much. I jumped on a plane and flew out to London.

It was a few weeks after your surgery. The last time I had seen you had been just after your second stroke, and you looked a lot better now. Rick got you out of bed and into a wheelchair for the first time. I think he wanted to remind you that there was a big world out there, just waiting for you.

They packed me up and wheeled me out, with my IV tubes, tracheostomy, respirator, my friend, and my nurses. They thought nothing of riding in a crowded elevator, walking down the hall to look at the flowers in the front lobby. We were going for an outing. It's all part of life in the Real World.

But the ICU is its own world: tiny, intense, and extremely limited. I would lie in my narrow white bed in my narrow white cubicle and have nightmares. I kept my eyes shut. There was nothing to see. I'd been in one hospital or another for a month and a half. To suddenly be out in a crowd was culture shock.

I couldn't handle all the motion. It was like an assault. I couldn't tell if I was moving or if other people were moving around me. If someone walked towards me, I felt like I was falling into them. And there were lots of people and they were all walking and they were either staring at me or going about their business trying not to. I saw myself out in the world for the first time in the lobby of that hospital, and I realized I was not normal. I was a Freak.

I had no control over my body, my mouth was hanging open, my hands were twisted and shaking. My legs were shamelessly jumping with clonus. A grim mental image rose in my mind, of pitiful creatures with their heads drooping and drooling. Vegetables. And I was one of them. That was me.

Anne Usher: You mouthed the word "freak." I felt awful that we hadn't thought about how you might react. You had trouble sitting up and you were tied into the chair, but as a nurse myself, I'm used to seeing tubes and machines and people flailing around. All I could see was how much better you were than you had been.

Michael: The ICU administration decided they needed your bed for somebody who was sicker. As soon as you were completely weaned off the respirator and onto the t-tube, they transferred you to the ward. It was all decided in the course of a few hours and then off you went, with no chance to say goodbye to Rick or Mary.

Unlike the ICU, the ward was badly understaffed, with only two nurses per shift covering a large number of patients. During the day, they would come into your room periodically, and turn and suction you on a schedule that fit in with all their other tasks. It was not great.

But at night it was much worse. The head nurse thought you were demanding, neurotic, and taking too much of his time. When he handled you he was rough and abrupt, never talking to you, or explaining what he was doing. Every time that nurse walked in the room, you flinched.

The panic attacks got worse. His response was to pump you full of Valium, which was prescribed for you as a PRN— to be used as required at the nurse's discretion. He said the best way of dealing with you would be for me to go away and leave it to him. I was considered part of the problem as if, by taking your fears seriously, I was contributing to your "neurosis."

After two days on the ward I said, "We might as well go home to Montreal." Even if the care was no better at the JGH, as a member of the hospital staff I could at least do a better job of manipulating the system.

I remember Skip Peerless' last rounds, the day I left London, three weeks after my surgery. I thanked him for the hundredth time and then I asked The Question. The question I had been too sick and then too scared to ask. "When will I be well again?" I fumbled with the letter board in my nervousness and in the end Michael had to read my lips.

"I'd guess you'll be standing by Thanksgiving and walking by Christmas," Skip answered. Standing by Thanksgiving: less than a month. Walking by Christmas: three months. It became my mantra. Repeated by Michael and all my friends: "Standing by Thanksgiving, walking by Christmas."

For now it was time to go home.

JEWISH GENERAL HOSPITAL

❋ Back at the JGH ❋

Night after night, all night.

Pt awake and agitated. Pt flailing both arms over head. Pt asking to have husband called.

I couldn't move my legs. I was trapped in the sheets. My arm was falling through the slats of the guardrail, flattening and stretching, like Elastic Man or Rubber Man, some guy from Seth's old superhero comic books. Mr. Fantastic, that's it. My whole body was going to be flattened and squished through the bed rails until I strangled. The nurse was mad at me.

Pt demanding attention. Given Xanax. Ludiomil. Haldol.

Michael: You were racked with panics every night. You were nearly delirious from lack of sleep. And the nurses, shortstaffed as they were, had a hard time dealing with you.

The Hun was the worst. She thought the panic attacks were a bunch of nonsense and I should pull myself together and stop being a baby. It didn't help that she had a German accent. She evoked all the deep-seated Jewish fears and prejudices about Germans that were surfacing in my nightmares. She had such power over me. She was there after everyone left for the night. Every day I would ask Michael if she was on duty, and I'd beg him not to leave me if she was. I used to fear Michael alienating her, that she would take it out on me after he left.

Michael: I was very angry with her one day and I said, "You know, I notice that you do much better with comatose patients. I bet you prefer them." And she said to me, "You're right, I do."

Patricia was still there in the bed next to mine! She was still in a coma and her husband was still sitting by her bed talking to her. Michael would talk to me and J.P. would talk to Patricia. "*Ma chere. Ma fille. Ma belle que j'adore. Ma belle marie.*" They must have been in their fifties, but he kept talking about her as a young and beautiful girl, his bride. Had there really been a time when I thought her good-as-dead and him a fool? Now I knew she was listening, as I was listening. We were rooting for each other.

Suzi Scott: The whole time Patricia was in High-Care, she never even blinked. Then one evening, J.P. comes running up to me and says, "Suzi, she talked!" And I think, "Oh yeah, I'll believe anything." But he says, "No, no, Suzi, you have to come see." So I go over and sure enough, her eyes are open and she's mouthing the words, "*Je t'aime.* I love you." J.P. starts crying. I start crying. "She's back! She's back!"

My right leg was still completely paralyzed. Every day the doctors stuck pins in my toes and shook their heads. I was still tube fed and incontinent. I wasn't having much success with the bedpan. There was a green, plasticized pad underneath me, which used to get all bunched up and stuck to my body. It reminded me of the diapers I used to put on Mom. For peeing I had a catheter and bag. My vagina and rectum were sore. Everything was sore. They wiped me with some kind of cloth that felt like sandpaper to my heightened sensitivity.

Everyone said I was improving. I graduated from bed baths to tub baths. The orderly wheeled me down a long corridor to an endless row of tiny bathtub rooms. In my mind it stretched out for miles. Then he would park me beside a big winching machine, and the nurse would take my gown off and wrap me, diaper-fashion, in a rubber sling attached to cables. Then the orderly would turn on the machine. It would start up with a horrible grinding sound, and lift me into the air. I would hang there, my limp body like a stunned fish in a net. I think my eyes were closed. I have no memory of the bathtub below me, the nurse standing by to guide me down. *The grinding went on and on, and then the warm water closed around my body. The water stroked me, soothed me, terrified me. I knew I didn't have the strength to keep my head from going under. I heard someone scream-ing; maybe it was me. The nurse bathed and shampooed me. Then there was the shower sound. The screaming and the shower; the bald Nazi, the concentration camp.*

The days hung on Michael's visits. No matter how mis-treated I felt or how awful the panics were, I knew it would be better when Michael came. Michael would put me to bed every night. He would read to me, and stroke me and breathe with me until I dozed off.

Michael: Your panics kept getting worse. I was at my wits' end. I asked Bernard to resume your acupuncture treat-ments. You were calmer after seeing him, but only temporarily. I asked Michael and Lesley to come in. I im-plored my psychiatrist friend, Laurence Kirmayer, to work with you, even though he had largely given up clinical psy-chiatry for research. I went to the NFB and explained the panic attacks and asked your friends to come see you.

I was exhausted, but it was nothing compared to what you were going through. People kept telling me I should go see a shrink. But that wasn't what I needed; I needed you to get better.

I got my support from colleagues at Herzl. The nurses, the doctors, the secretaries. They looked after me. I had started seeing a few patients again at this point. Cheryl Levitt had taken over as Acting Director. Some days I would just walk into Cheryl's office and say, "I'm not coping." She never talked much, or asked questions. She would just sit down and hold my hand.

Cheryl Levitt: I remember one night I dropped by High-Care on my way home, and walked into the middle of a panic attack. I was terrified. I'd never seen anyone going through that. Your eyes opened up and you had these weird, spastic movements of your hand. You were mouthing words but there was no sound. You were asking me to get Michael. But when I called him, he said "I have to sleep. Just for a few hours and then I'll come."

I felt terrible, because I wanted him there nearly as desperately as you did, but he was at the end of his strength. So I said to you, "I don't think Michael can come in, but I'll stay with you for a while." I couldn't leave because the nurse on shift was someone you were scared of. You were panicking for nearly an hour and a half before you fell asleep. Nothing seemed to help. You kept mouthing the words "I want to die. I want to die."

I don't remember asking to die, but it's there in the nurses' notes too. I don't think it meant I wanted to commit suicide or wished someone would do it for me. It meant: I hurt, I'm scared, get me out of here.

Kathleen Shannon: We had worked together for years at Studio D, but we weren't close. You always radiated a kind of cheerful confidence, as if you had your life just the way you wanted it. I wasn't exactly jealous, it just never occurred to me that you would need anything from me. Then Michael came to the film board and asked us to visit.

When I walked into your cubicle, it was hard to tell whether you were greeting me with delight or freaking out. Your body was speaking a whole other language that I had never seen before. Your facial expression was all untuned.

It struck me that it would be stressful for you to have to welcome me, or entertain me. So I said, "I'm just going to keep you company while you rest. Don't worry about saying anything; you can say it later." I stroked your arm and kept telling you, "Don't worry about anything, everything can wait." You seemed to fall asleep at that point, but then someone else dropped by and you got all anxious trying to be understood by them.

Michael: It soon became apparent that this chaos of visitors was only adding to your anxiety. We needed to create a delicate balance between your need for rest and your need for company. Sara Lazzam, my secretary, started setting up a schedule where you would see only one person at a time, for half an hour. Each morning she would create a list of the day's visitors for you.

I loved Sara's schedules. I don't know if I ever thanked her enough for the diplomacy it required to retract "appointments" from the people I decided I didn't want to see. I quickly learned who gave me energy and who drained me. Conversations with anyone but Michael or Naomi or Seth were exhausting and sometimes ridiculous. Michael says I usually communicated sympathy for folks who couldn't understand me, but in truth I was sick of the letter board. Often when someone correctly guessed the letter I was trying to point to, they would jump to conclusions about the rest of the word and even finish my sentence on the basis of that one letter. I watched in helpless frustration as the game of charades spun out of control in the wrong direction.

Michael: The reason you couldn't talk wasn't because you couldn't remember or access language, as happens sometimes with hemispheric strokes. It was because, for a while, you were unable to breathe. One needs breath to speak, and your breath was being provided through a tube in your throat. The major concern of the neurologists was to protect your airway, and the fact that you couldn't talk with a tracheostomy was considered to be a temporary state that I shouldn't get excited about. I, on the other hand, was very concerned about your ability to talk, especially in light of your panic attacks. I was trying to bridge the importance of the medical concerns, which I didn't deny, with your psychological well-being.

The solution was to decrease the size of the trach tube, so the opening gradually got smaller and smaller. Then you could cover the trach tube with your thumb, for short phrases.

Seth: I was home for the weekend the first time you spoke. I don't remember what you said; I just have this picture in my mind of Dad's hand covering the trach tube, and you making noise through your mouth. And then you smiled. It was a tremendous relief. We're all big talkers in our family.

Pt is learning how to cover her trach to communicate w. voice. She needs some direction as to where it is. The closure she maintains is adequate for intelligible voice. Should this not be possible, a nurse may cover the trach for her. She needs to be reminded to take a deep breath before closing.

The first sounds were breathy, less than whispers. My Jackie Kennedy voice, Terre called it. The therapists called

it "not functional." It was hard work. I learned the economics of speech. To measure my words, as the cliché goes.
When it's so difficult to get ideas across, most of them seem
hardly worth it. A lot of self-censorship occurred: "Never
mind, it's not important."

The speech therapist said that I would never regain normal speech. I could try, and she could help, but we were
doomed to failure. The damage had been done, and we had
to be "realistic" in our expectations. She was cool and brisk,
as if she had just stopped off at the hospital on the way to
doing something really important, like preparing to give a
dinner party.

I was devastated. How could I be me if I couldn't speak?
Who the hell did she think she was? Who taught her it was
her job to make me "realistic," to dash my so-called false
hopes? I *was* talking! Real words. I had no strength to
project them, but they were all there. Or mostly there. I
could only get out a few words at a time, so my phrasing
was weird and irregular. My thick tongue made my words
slurred and people had trouble understanding me. I had to
repeat everything as I became more fatigued. Requests came
out as baby talk or one-word commands: "Radio," not
"Would you please turn on the radio?" Sometimes I grunted.
But it just wasn't conceivable that this weak voice would
not strengthen with time and practice.

I can't remember the speech therapist ever coming after
that. Maybe she just gave up on this hopeless case. I don't
think she did any speech exercises with me, not even the
tongue movements and clicks I had done after the first

stroke. And she never had the decency to admit I was doing better than she had predicted, or to congratulate me.

I didn't know why I had trouble speaking, that the stroke had damaged my cranial nerves, paralyzing one vocal cord and half my tongue and palate. Michael says he knew, and maybe he told me but I didn't understand.

I talked slowly because I was thinking slowly and my breath was slow. I wasn't able to be glib and just rattle things off like I used to. But some people really listened. They had to be quiet to hear me. There's something compelling about such speech, something sacred in the silences.

My hearing was painfully acute. I could hear people whispering about me from the nursing station across the ICU, or at least I thought it was about me. I recognized everyone's different footsteps. Loud voices frightened me. The paging system was the worst—intrusive and insensitive, going about its business in flat tones as if we weren't sick and sometimes dying. "Dr. Swift to the ICU! Dr. Swift, stat!"

I would become confused and overwhelmed if I was supposed to do two things at the same time, like have my lips swabbed with glycerin and listen to a conversation. If there was talking, there could be no music; if there was music, there could be no talking. I couldn't separate them into channels, as I had without thinking before my stroke. Now I became the music that I heard; there were no boundaries. I could follow all the various instruments, as if I were inside the heads of the composer and the musicians, participating in their creation. I would laugh at a trumpet improvising, or nod to a flute responding to cello. But anything with a strong beat was painful. The rhythms pounded in my whole being. Ladysmith Black Mambazo, my favorite group from the summer before, became scary. Orchestral extravaganzas and Renaissance fanfares were frantic. Opera was too noisy. Violins were too shrill. I became addicted to Mozart and Glenn Gould's rendition of the *Goldberg Variations,* as well as some New Age music that I had previously scorned. Environmental tapes of running streams and bird sounds were mainlined through earphones to create my own private island on the hospital bed. The cliché was true: music soothed my frayed nervous system.

The nose tube went through my nose all the way down to my stomach, and it irritated the whole tract. My throat was always sore. I would pull the tube out, usually in the middle of the night. I'm not sure if I was pulling it out on purpose or in my sleep. I remember one of the nurses yelling at me, "Bad girl! You pulled out your tube!" She wasn't allowed to put it back in, so she had to call the neurology resident. And of course I couldn't eat meanwhile, so the dietitian would be there scolding me about dehydration and malnutrition.

Reinsertion was painful, probably because I pulled it out so often. I remember exactly what it felt like. It goes down your throat and into your esophagus, and then you have to kind of swallow it down. I would always ask for Michael to reinsert my feeding tube because he was so gentle and smooth with it. It was the resident's job, but if he didn't come, Michael would just do it.

I was a perfectly terrible patient, a royal pain in the ass, and so was Michael.

The hospital was short on nurses, short on orderlies. They couldn't turn me at my discomfort, they had to turn by the clock. No one seemed to know the "sheet trick" the London nurses had used so it was an awkward procedure. Each time I was turned, they also had to "position" me, wedging me into an elaborate nest of pillows. I felt like a flower arrangement or maybe a corpse. I lacked the control to lie on my side unsupported without flopping over. There was one pillow in front to keep me from rolling, one doubled up against my back, and one between my legs. I used to beg to be repositioned because I would get numb at the pressure points. My body was a dead weight and I didn't know where my limbs were. But I had trouble remembering the word "position." I would ask for "posturing" or "placing" or "set-up." Exact words often eluded me, forcing me to invent approximations.

Gerry Rogers: I remember on my first visit, going up the elevator, so afraid to see you. The first thing you said to me was, "Hi, I missed your birthday." You were smiling but kind of shaky, and your eyes were rolling around. You were desperately skinny, like a concentration camp survivor, and your muscles were like jelly. One arm kept floating off in the air, and you would say, "No control." This was going to be the first night when Michael wouldn't be sitting with you until you fell asleep. I would be there instead. It was a big deal and we were all nervous. You were so afraid that you weren't going to be able to sleep, but you kept saying, "Michael has to rest."

Pt coughing up thick yellow mucous. Pt restless and noisy.
Pt really demanding, wants to change position every 30 min.
Given Haldol.

One panic melted into the next. I begged the nurse to
untangle my legs from the sheets but she was busy charting. They were always charting.

Annie sang me a lullaby to help me sleep; something
about flying, one of my favorites. She used to sing that same
song to Seth and then Naomi. She always sang it with hand
gestures, in a soft voice:

My pigeon house (fingers interlocked)
I open wide, (hands twist, fingers unlock)
And set my pigeons free. (fingers fluttering ...)
They climb so high
Till they reach the sky
And they light on the nearest tree ...
Ku-ru, Ku-ru
Ku-ru, ku-ru, ku-ru.

I was the baby now. That was OK. It was good.

Annie Klein: I sang "My Pigeon House" for you, and when
I got to the Ku-ru's, you sang with me. It was soon after
they fixed your trach so you could talk a bit, and your voice
was so sweet. I'll always remember that.

Pt confused, waving her arms about. Haldol 0.5 mg.

I hated that I had missed Rosh Hashanah. It's a time to
reflect, reevaluate life and make resolves for the coming

year; a time to appreciate life and its blessings. We had always celebrated with my mother—she would come from Philadelphia for the High Holy Days and for Passover, even before she came to live with us.

One of the few good things about being back at the JGH was that Jewish holidays were acknowledged. Two men came around to blow the shofar just after sundown on Yom Kippur, the Day of Atonement. I loved the idea that they were coming to me because I couldn't go to synagogue. But the wild, primeval notes quickly became too shrill for my super-sensitive ears. I anxiously waved them away.

My leg was stuck in the bed rails. My bad leg that Bernard said wasn't "bad," only lethargic. My body was infinitely distortable. It was squished flat. It was a melted soda bottle. I called and called with my weak voice. I banged on the bedframe, over and over, with my numb fists.

In the morning I noticed that my knuckles were blue.

❧ Interlude: Restraints ❧

Journal: July 3, 1990, Black Lake
I was lying in bed just now, for an afternoon read with Robin Morgan's *Dry Your Smile*. The narrator was describing her mother's violent attack on her under the influence of L-Dopa. The hospital staff rushed in and put her in restraints. RE-STRAINTS! I shot up in bed like in bad movies. The memory of restraints washed over me. I cried out, sobbed, shook, wanted

Michael. I'm amazed that with all my remembering, this particular horror has not come back to me until now, almost three years after the stroke, and has come back with all its original terror. I fear that I will have this kind of flashback forever. For the first few years, a smell, a sound, a phrase would trigger vivid replays of painful events. But beyond the pain, there is a deep relief in exhuming these memories.

I remember the feeling more than the details. I am at the JGH, in a panic attack and thrashing to pull out a tube—is it the tracheostomy or the nasal feeding tube? In my panic, I grab at one of the nurses or aides, begging her not to leave me, and she gets scared or angry. Orderlies are called to restrain me. I think they just use pieces of sheeting, tying each of my hands to the bed rails. I continue to thrash, my paralysis now exaggerated by this physical leashing. I feel like a prisoner. But no, I must be crazy—this is a reliable hospital. The staff must be acting appropriately. I wondered before if the panic attacks meant that I was going crazy, and now I think they do.

I don't know how often I was put in restraints. I only know that I lived in fear of them. I remember being threatened with them if I didn't behave, if I pulled out the tubes. They were the "or else."

My family seemed to know nothing of this part of my experience; it happened at night after Michael had left. But the medical notes tell the story.

Pt needs to be restrained ...
Wrist restraints applied for safety so the pt will not pull at her trach or feeding tube ...
Pt sleeping quietly, arm restraints removed....

❧ Screamer ❧

I remember a voice. A woman howling, "Nurse, nurse, help me, somebody help me. Don't leave me alone." It went on and on. Her voice ripped me apart. It was as if I were inside her body. I could have been her. Sometimes I was her.

People crying, walking around drugged out and drooling: I got used to it, like the nurses were used to it. "She's just a screamer, don't bother about her. We have a few on every ward." Who was this new self who could hear someone beg for help and accept the nurse's verdict that it was "nothing?"

∼

My limbs were numb and distant, like strange objects lying in my bed. I remember the soft rubbery texture under my fingers. *This is not my skin.* I remember my hands spasming into claws, fingernails digging into my flesh, leaving marks that I couldn't feel. *I remember Mom digging marks into her hands because they didn't keep her nails short. I would cut her nails and try to stretch her fingers out, but it would hurt her. Finally I had to accept that her fingers couldn't be straightened.*

Joe Carlton: You asked me if you were going crazy and I said no, you were hypersensitive. Small things seemed life threatening. It was understandable. Often it's only after a crisis has begun to resolve that one can really look at what is happening. It's then that we are most susceptible to terror.

Eventually Michael persuaded the hospital to hire sit-ters overnight so someone would always be at my bedside to help with my panics. It was an awful job, I knew that. I felt like I was imposing on them, asking these underpaid women to stay awake and take care of me. You can't pay somebody to love you. But the people who loved me were already strained to the limit.

Every night I'd somehow ask the sitter to pat my head. It was a hypnotic motion that calmed me down and helped me sleep. It was very awkward. Why was I asking a total stranger to do this weird and intimate thing? Often I would outlast her ability to keep patting without falling asleep herself.

I remember asking one woman to read from Kahlil Gibran's *The Prophet*. She was a francophone who could hardly speak English, let alone read this convoluted, ar-chaic translation. She stumbled through it, missing words and fracturing phrases. I felt ashamed to put her through that, but I was desperate for the words.

23:45   Pt can't fall asleep. Wants to die. Attempted to reassure.
Pt asked us to kill her, wants to stop breathing.
Haldol 1 mg.

Seth: Your stroke entirely transformed my relationship with Naomi. She and I hadn't been very close in high school. We fought about all the things teenagers fight about: the telephone, her sloppiness. I thought she was a screw-up. I didn't understand her at all.

Naomi: If someone had told me in grade eleven that I was going to be living alone with my father the next year, I would have jumped off a cliff. There was no way. He and I were at each other's throats. It was a power struggle and I always lost. Mom was the mediator for everything that happened in that house. When she would go on location with some film, I would go crazy.

But after everyone came back from London, it was just me and Dad. Suddenly, we were a family. The two of us. He needed me. And he knew that he needed me. The power struggle was over. When you need someone, you're much more careful with the way you treat them.

Naomi had begun Brébeuf, a classy academic *cégep* (Quebec's junior college system) in the French-from-France tradition. Most of the students had attended private French secondary school. Naomi's French, while fluent and colloquial, was purely Québecois, learned at a populist summer camp. Seth had gone to Brébeuf for a year before going on the SAGE tour and he had survived, but Naomi was drowning there.

Naomi: By the time classes started, my mother was in the hospital and I was the walking wounded, an open sore. This was supposed to be a challenge, but I wasn't up for it. My French, which was considered stellar at my English high school, was a disaster.

I couldn't meet people. I walked around the school on the verge of tears. Brébeuf is two blocks from the JGH and I shuttled back and forth so many times a day that it seemed like the two buildings were attached.

I don't know when I stopped going to classes. I convinced myself somehow that I had dropped out, that it was official. The only problem was that I didn't tell anyone. Every day that I missed, my teachers were busy giving me zeros on assignments that I didn't even know I had. I "officially" left Brébeuf at the end of the term. The highest mark I got was a 16 percent.

Naomi spared me this information. Instead, she told amusing anecdotes, and I chose to be proud of her going to such a tough school. Once she said she wanted to quit because she was doing badly, but I brushed it off saying surely they would understand and she probably wasn't doing as badly as she thought.

All I knew was that I was dependent on Naomi, and she was my unfailing confidante and advocate. But it was a difficult position for a seventeen year old. Lacking any status in the hospital, she would do her best to shield me from the Hun and anyone else who mistreated me. After all those years of trying to teach her to be "nicer" to adults, I now needed her to protect me against them.

Naomi: Suzi Scott and I ganged up on my captive mother and did a complete beauty makeover. I had my mother wearing more makeup in the hospital than she would wear to an awards banquet. I had always desperately wanted her to look like one of the suburban Hampstead moms. This was my chance, I suppose. My friends whom my family had always dismissed as useless airheads came in to do facial masks, even lip treatments. We were useful for the first time. Thank God for *Seventeen Magazine*.

Naomi had spent years locked in the bathroom, valuable years when (I thought) she should have been acquiring the skills and competence she would need as a female in this society. Math. Sports. Automobile mechanics. Instead she was becoming an expert in hair color and make up. Her feminist mother and her doctor father both managed to miss the fact that her bathroom hibernation also included long bouts of bulimia.

For Naomi to swab apricot balm on my parched lips, to bleach the dark hairs on my face (the result of those misprescribed steroids), to do something as intimate as shave my armpits, sounds natural between mother and daughter. Hadn't I wiped her sweet baby bum, combed her little-girl braids, nursed the bumps and bruises of body and heart? But daughters—and mothers—forget, and it had been so long since we were comfortable with each other's bodies. She wore a loose sweatshirt for the entire year in which she grew secret breasts, and demanded that I not make a "big deal" when she informed me that she had begun menstruating at camp.

So it was doubly—no, triply—sweet to share Naomi's new Sultry Peach lipstick. My skin was blotched, my features lopsided, my limbs slack and wasted, but my daughter made me feel pretty.

I remember the smell of her hands stroking my face during an anxiety attack. It must have been hard for her to watch me twitching and gasping, but she never pulled away.

≈

I felt confused and betrayed when Suzi Scott announced she was now Wanda the Witch. I guess she thought she was being cute, but I had no sense of humor about it. Suzi was the only nurse who loved me, and now she had decided to get tough with me. She refused to untangle me when my nightgown attacked my legs. She said I should learn to wait. She refused to help me find CBC on my bedside radio. She said I could do it myself. Why now? Had I done something wrong? Was she only pretending to like me?

Seth had given me that radio to keep me connected with the real world, the world outside the hospital. CBC was all I listened to, but somehow it always seemed to be tuned to some Top 40 station. I had great difficulty learning how to operate that simple machine—not just physical but mental. There were countless hours of having to listen to the wrong station, with annoying commercials and brainless deejay banter piped directly into my brain through the earphones.

Suzi Scott: When you started to be able to move your fingers, that's when I started playing with your radio. Once a day I would move the dial as far from CBC as possible. It was a way to get you to use your hands. You needed to realize you could do things for yourself. I think you knew I was doing it, because you used to call me "Bitch." It took you awhile, but you learned to change the station.

Panics continued to come suddenly and without provocation. I would be with a visitor and suddenly feel like I couldn't swallow and was going to choke and die. I seemed to be on a million different drugs, which confirmed my fear that I was going mad. Fortunately the psychologists from Herzl were my friends, people who knew me when I was OK, who thought I would be OK again. Michael had asked them to help me with daily relaxation exercises. I remember Yvonne's hypnotic voice counting backwards. Judy had me visualize ocean waves. Morrie added gestures: tapping my left hand, which was more spastic, with my right one as I was saying "Calm. Relax." There was deep breathing associated with it. Breathe in relaxation. Breathe out tension and fear.

As soon as I felt the shortness of breath, the constricting chest, I would start the exercise: calm, relax, calm, relax, ten, nine, eight . . . I struggled to remember the exact words and motions. Breathe in—inspiration? Breathe out—what? Perspiration? If I got it right, perhaps it would save me.

Morrie Golden: The words didn't matter. You needed some sense of active participation, of control. If it was a full-blown attack that had already overtaken you, then nothing would work. But I remember watching the panic start to roll over you, and you take hold and diminish it.

Many of the High-Care staff didn't take what we were doing very seriously. Sometimes I would show up for our appointment and the nurse would say, "This is not visiting hours." And I would say "This isn't a visit." But as far as she was concerned, we were just chatting. It wasn't important enough to write on your chart. It wasn't hardcore medicine like drugging you would be.

Laurence Kirmayer: In the end, Haldol may have been part of the problem, rather than part of the solution. It's not a good drug for anxiety; it can add to your disorientation. It can cause odd symptoms, like stiffness, drifting arms, and phantom limb stuff. But it's a very common medication, and probably used too often with unclear or minor rationale.

You seemed to be displaying those typical Haldol side effects, so I wrote a note on your chart asking that Haldol be avoided if possible, and suggesting Cogentin to counteract some of the side effects. But I was just a consulting psychiatrist—it would have been up to the attending neurologist to write the orders. That night you had an extremely bad time and were given the full dose of Haldol. The next day I left a stronger note, recommending that Haldol be discontinued. It was replaced with chloral hydrate, for treating your sleeplessness rather than some supposed psychosis.

How long had it been since I had a real night's sleep? Two weeks? Three? Michael decided that maybe if I didn't nap during the day and stayed awake well into the evening, I might be able to reestablish a normal sleeping pattern. That made theoretical sense, but in practice it was horrendous. My entire roster of visitors was recruited to keep me from dozing. Again and again I would start to drift off, only to be forced awake. Michael would program my evenings, trying to keep me entertained while I waited for the hour when I was finally allowed to shut my eyes. He would lift me from the bed and wheel me downstairs to the Herzl conference room. There he would project some of the family slides he had assembled after the first stroke. After the slide show came the telephone. Michael would pull out my little phone book and say, "Who shall we call tonight?" I usually had enough energy to make one call. It was like a game: Michael would dial and hold the receiver for me and I would surprise the hell out of somebody.

I remember calling Norma, my college roommate, who lives in Boston. I said, "Hello, Norma? This is Bonnie," and she started crying. The next night we called Razelle. She screamed. "It's my sister! I've got my sister back." I understood for the first time the extent of her fear of losing me.

Phone calls seemed to require even more vocal projection than talking in person, and I was self-conscious about my lengthy pauses, knowing there was a long distance bill to pay. But they would leave me feeling happy and loved, ready for my bed and a good night's sleep—which would last all of a few hours before it was panic time again.

02:00   pt noisy & confused.
        States she had "bad dream" where she was "paralyzed."

Gerry Rogers: I brought a floral brocade writing book to the hospital for your visitors to write in. I called it *The Friends' Book of Healing.* I thought, "Recovery is going to be slow, and probably the hardest thing for Bonnie will be to remember how bad it was and realize what a big victory each new movement is." The changes were so apparent to us on the outside and yet for you it was like a sea without markers of time and space and change.

My other thought was that probably some people wanted to say things to you but weren't quite able to say them out loud, so the book would be a safe place to communicate. In the back of my mind, I was also thinking that if you didn't pull through, then this would be really precious to your kids and Michael.

The Friends' Book of Healing:
You told me this is the "improvements" book—so, this being my first visit, I've got to say you are a lot better than I thought you'd be—such good smiles—and much activity with your arms and lots of secretions, which you're spitting into recycled tissue. Love you a lot. Try to be calm—better times will come, and we'll be bitching together in the halls of the NFB.

Love, Gloria

It was a funny time. On the one hand, I was constantly anxious; on the other, I felt bathed in love. My hospital room was a melting pot where Catholic nuns met feminist witches, and physicians met acupuncturists and deep muscle massage therapists. I remember watching one of my NFB friends in animated discussion with Ron and wondering, "Does she know he's a rabbi? Does he know she's a lesbian?" It was gloriously mixed up.

The stroke had restored my love and faith in men, erased my knee-jerk prejudices that were an easy but unnecessary side effect of the pain of sexism. My women's networks had rallied around me, from sacred rites on the mountain and inventing *The Friends' Book of Healing,* to domestic details like bringing me real food and nurturing my family. I had a special closeness with women who were mothers during my worst weeks. They were at ease with my physical helplessness, they knew how to dress me, feed me. But I couldn't separate my women friends from the men who also formed my "net" in this crisis. Until my stroke, Michael and Seth had been the only "exceptions" allowed into my women-centered life. But now my life embraced gentle healers like Joe Carlton, Rabbi Ron, Rick; Bob Usher who cried with joy at the foot of my wheelchair; male film colleagues whom I had previously excluded from my "inner circle" but who were brave enough to include themselves in my healing; Bernard, who was there almost daily and ended every acupuncture session with a kiss—it was part of the treatment.

❋ Turning Point ❋

The Friends' Book of Healing:
> *Every time I come, you keep looking better—calm and relaxed. Now you're sitting up and getting ready to go to the gym. If you could just get that tube out of your nose!*
> *All in good time—as Kohelet said, "To everything there is a season and a time for every purpose under heaven." Now is the time for healing.*
> *Love, Ron Aigen*

What changed? It was probably a combination of factors: stopping Haldol, relaxation exercises, Michael's forced wakefulness regimen, the simple passage of time. According to the medical notes it happened very quickly; one night was solid terror, the next night was broken and restless, and the next was smooth sleep with a single short-lived nightmare at dawn.

Being able to sleep brought an immediate turnaround on all other fronts. Each day was a benchmark. Suzi Scott taught me to turn myself, carefully isolating each step in the process. First I had to reach for the metal bed rail; then, using my arm strength which was greater than that of my legs or trunk, I had to wriggle myself face-down on the bed. Then, after a rest, I could reach with the other arm for the other side of the bed and slowly worm the rest of my body over until I was facing the other way.

This exercise was complicated by the piles of pillows that kept me in place. I didn't have the strength to move them out of my way, let alone set them up for my new position. I couldn't distinguish my own limbs from the pillows, and often floundered around trying to rearrange or remove my legs. Suzi wouldn't help me until I had completed all the steps I was capable of, and struggled for a while with the ones I wasn't. It was a Big Moment when I rolled over entirely by myself. No more waiting on the every-two-hours schedule.

I started physio again, with Iolanda. It was grueling work. I don't know if I can adequately describe the fatigue: it was profound, blinding, literally unspeakable. When fatigue hit I could no longer form words in my mind or my mouth. I stammered and my tongue got in the way. All my new skills deserted me and I cried for my bed.

I remember collapsing in misery when I tried and tried but still couldn't lift my right leg; when I couldn't sit unsupported on my gym platform; when I couldn't get my toothbrush into my mouth but smeared toothpaste across my face for the millionth time. Iolanda would counter my despair by reminding me of all the things I now took for granted—like breathing—and how hard they had once been.

Learning to use the bedpan was a long and complicated process. It had been months since peeing was something I decided to do rather than something that happened to me. I had lost the ability to recognize when I needed to go.

Kathleen Shannon: All the rules of privacy that people keep between each other had changed. One time we were talking very seriously about film board politics and you suddenly said, "I'm shitting," and asked me to get the bedpan. I kind of blew it because I didn't move fast enough and I didn't know how to slide the bedpan under you. In fact I failed entirely, and you shit in the bed—very tidily, I must say. I stood there with the bedpan in my hand, wondering how to clean you up. I felt embarrassed at my embarrassment. I would have liked to have taken everything in my stride.

Gerry Rogers: One time when I came to visit, you were sitting up in the chair, showing off your new exercises. I remember your feeding tube was hanging down from your nose and every now and then as you were talking you would pick it up and swing it around and we would both crack up. Hospital humor.

But then you started to get tired. You told me: "I want to get in bed, I have to get in bed." I went and asked the nurse and she rang for the orderly, but he didn't come. You were starting to shake from sitting there, because sitting up was still a hard thing for you.

Finally, the orderly came in and without saying a word
he swooped you out of your chair and plunked you on the
bed. It was almost violent. Then he walked out the door,
without even looking at you. I thought I should say something to Michael about it, and then I thought, "No. When
you are dependent like that, if you alienate any of the staff
you are really helpless." The main thing I could see that
would help, was for you to get out of that place.

When Michael told me that I would probably go to a
rehabilitation institute after I left hospital, I thought he
meant to rest up before diving back into normal life.

The only Anglophone rehab institute was way out in
the suburb of Chomedy where I would be isolated from my
friends and family. So Michael applied to the Institut de
Réadaptation de Montréal, a French institution, founded
by Dr. Gustav Gingras, after he became internationally famous for his rehabilitation of Korean war veterans.

Iolanda described it as summer camp, a live-in gym run
by the physios. Summer camp was my favorite childhood
place. I was euphoric.

But the Institut only accepted people who stood to gain
by rehabilitation. If you were too far gone, you were doomed
to stay that way. If "they" believed there was room for
improvement, you were accepted. Plus you had to have
reached a certain level of independence to be admitted. Nose
tubes and tracheostomies did not meet their dress code.
The scarce beds came up only rarely and unpredictably,
and when they came, you had to be ready.

Naomi: My dad was losing his mind because they couldn't find a bed in a rehab institute and he didn't think that my mom was getting sufficient physio at the JGH. He felt like we were losing time. One morning my dad and I were having breakfast in the kitchen and he started talking about bringing Mom home. He said we could put a hospital bed in the dining room, have round-the-clock home nursing and therapists visiting the house. He wanted to set up an ICU in our dining room. He was back at work full time at this point and really wanted everything to return to normal. As if Mom being home would mean everything was OK. I got really mad, telling him I didn't want an ICU in the dining room, that I had to go to school and everything. I was chain-smoking boyfriends at that time: one after another with some very messy overlaps. I was very needy and my judgment was sometimes a little off. Dad made me feel like I was incredibly selfish, like I didn't care. We had a huge fight, and I remember telling him that no matter what happened, I was never going to have my mother again in the same way. I felt the loss of a comfort, a net, of some level of childhood that I had been planning to hold onto for a few more years. Of course I cared. He eventually dropped the idea of moving my mom home just yet.

I worked like crazy to learn the skills I needed to be admitted to the Institut. Iolanda taught me how to use a wheelchair. My tendency was to go in circles since my right arm was much stronger than my left. I wheeled into furniture and scraped my knuckles. Stopping was not an automatic reflex any more than pushing the wheels. More often than not, I ran into walls to stop myself.

My wheelchair didn't have footrests, probably in order

to give my legs more exercise. So I would be "walking" as I wheeled: a slow process with my left foot struggling to keep up and my right foot dragging unwillingly along the floor.

I would get breathless fast. My little coordination disappeared with fatigue till I was going round and round in circles of frustration. But how proud I was, the first time I pushed through a doorway without marking the walls.

I was determined to learn to swallow. I needed to be off the feeding tube. Besides, I missed the pure pleasure of eating. When the sickeningly rich smell of the supplement seeped through the nose tube and into my brain, I fantasized about water: clear, delicious, amazing water. I felt cheated because I had missed the fruits of late summer— raspberries, peaches, tomatoes, and Annie's sweet corn.

According to the medical notes, my first real food was a few spoonfuls of apple sauce and puréed carrots administered by one of the physios. My trach secretions were "rosy" after that, showing that I hadn't been able to swallow the carrots, but had inhaled them instead. I was told I couldn't expect to achieve a "functional swallow" until my breathing was declared out of danger and my trach tube was removed. That night I pulled out the trach tube in my sleep.

Suzi Scott: The trach tube is like a piece of plastic with a hollow finger that's inserted into a hole in your throat. You were off the respirator by that point, but the tube was still in your throat to keep the hole open and allow the suction catheter to be passed in and out. When the tube is removed, the hole closes and scar tissue forms, and then if the patient has to be reintubated, it's a problem. So until everybody is confident that the patient isn't going to have any respiratory problems, it just stays in, tied to the side with a ribbon. But you got tired of it and I think you just untied the ribbon and popped it out. It was coming out eventually, but you were ready and you just took charge. There was a lot of shaking of heads and clicking of tongues, but in the end, they decided to jump the schedule and leave it out.

With my trach tube out, I was declared fit for serious eating practice, usually with a greyish purée of well-boiled vegetables from the hospital kitchen. At first I would gag back and spit out whatever I swallowed, but eventually it would stay down. I could only eat under staff supervision, because of the danger of choking. Luckily Michael passed for staff in this instance, and his ideas on nutrition were a little different. I'll never forget the super-thick coffee ice cream milkshake that was the first thing he fed me, stroking it down my throat to help me swallow. "Such naches," he said. Naches is Yiddish for well-deserved pleasures; "such naches" is used with ironic humor to note the tiny silver linings in immense storm clouds. It became a family code phrase.

After a while I graduated to beautiful mushed-up chicken and mashed potatoes that Meena sent from home, and small bits of solid food. I was drooling a lot and my hand-eye coordination was off. With half my mouth and tongue paralyzed, I couldn't feel when food dribbled on my face. People were always dabbing at me, and my nightgowns were filthy. It didn't bother me. Table manners were not a big issue at the time.

I was still on the feeding tube to supplement my nutrition, and I still pulled it out regularly. Finally, after I had pulled it out for the umpteenth time, the dietitian decided to leave it and work on getting enough food down me by mouth. I loved eating, but it was heavy exercise and I tired quickly. The dietitian posted a chart where my daily food intake was logged. I felt like a kid with a bad report card every time she came in to check it. She told me I was malnourished and that if I didn't increase my intake by the end of the week, she would order the resident to reinsert the feeding tube.

Learning to write was easier. Towards the end of October, the occupational therapist showed me how to grip a pencil, stabilize the paper, and rest my elbow on the tray table so my arm would be less spastic. It all went very fast, from squiggling to approximate her squares and circles in a broad and erratic way the first day, to copying them rather neatly the next day. Then I was writing whole words and sentences in a shaky kindergarten scrawl which betrayed my lack of fine motor skills. Everyone was impressed. I was a star.

The OT asked me to write a sentence a day, kind of like homework, but a sentence wasn't enough for me. My first attempt was a nearly illegible letter to Naomi.

At first I wrote on the loose pages the OT left me; then I asked Dorothy Hénaut for a journal of my own. Dorothy had been writing journals for as long as I knew her. I had always insisted that I had no time for that sort of thing, but now I began keeping one in earnest. It was more than an OT exercise. It was a tool for my survival. I was processing the strange and troubling events occurring in my body, recording thoughts I couldn't trust my damaged mind to remember, trying to make coherence out of chaos. Writing in my journal became as necessary a part of my daily routine as brushing my teeth and physical therapy.

Journal: October 23, 1987

Michael says my writing is already better than his. Today was very "up" with enormous changes in my movement. But now I am tired because I had company all day with no break. Several of my visitors remarked that now I look like the old Bonnie.

Journal: October 24, 1987

I had a session with Michele Devroede, my old psychotherapist. Laurence Kirmayer suggested I start seeing her again, since she had helped me during what we now know was a silent stroke, while I was filming the SAGE tour.

I hadn't seen her since we both went on vacation in August. When she walked in, I was so full of words I went into a major panic attack. She said, "It's OK, don't talk." She stood by my bed and held my numb feet for the whole hour. Her hands pressed hard against my soles, and both the numbness and the panic ebbed away. We stayed like that without talking for the whole session. I still remember how grounded I felt. How could she just walk in and devise exactly the right treatment?

Afterwards she explained that the panics could be the upper part of my body saying, "Whoa, wait a moment—there is no support underneath." She advised me to keep a pillow at the end of my bed for my feet to rest against. It's true—my upper body has progressed more quickly and has to wait for my legs to catch up. So the panic is a message—slow down and integrate. My own spirit has to put together all the separate therapies and progresses.

The move to the Institut was almost within my grasp. All my energy was focused towards that goal. So I was taken off guard one morning when Suzi told me I'd be going home for the weekend in a few days. At first I thought I must have misunderstood her. I could go home? Home to my own house? I told all my visitors this great news and how excited I was, but I didn't tell them the other part of it: I was scared to be leaving the hospital, even for a weekend. Was I ready? Would I be all right? Or was Michael pushing things again as he had that first night in the emergency room almost three months ago?

How could I get into our house, which had five big steps up to the front porch? How would I use the downstairs bathroom—a tiny converted closet with no room for a wheelchair? How would I get upstairs to our bedroom? It was all too frightening and too much trouble. I didn't belong there.

Michael, on the other hand, couldn't wait to get me

home. He had rented all sorts of hospital equipment—an IV hanger, a commode. I was overwhelmed by the extent of his desire to have me back. The tubes and machines and shitting in my pants were just petty details. I was his wife and he wanted me with him.

I remember that first ride home, in a special ambulance van with a lift for the wheelchair. My equilibrium was so unhinged that each bump in the road felt like a major accident. Every pebble was a cliff, every pothole a ravine. I couldn't tell what was moving: me or everything around me. When we drove down the street, my disordered senses said the buildings were falling sideways. When the attendants opened the van door, it felt like I was falling backwards. When they wheeled me out, it felt like the van was driving away. Michael reassured me that this sense of disorientation was all part of the stroke and would no doubt improve with time. That knowledge was comforting when I was safe in bed, but did nothing to lessen the terror of the experience as it was happening.

When we got to our high front steps, the attendants carried me up in the wheelchair. It was a heavy, awkward load. I worried that I would slip out of the chair or that my helpers would stumble and fall. With each lurch the steps seemed to fly up at me. Michael stood watching at the top of the stairs, his recurring back injury preventing him from grabbing me out of their hands, but not from yelling anxious instructions. I was home.

Once I was inside my family conspired to turn obstacles into adventures. Seth, who had greatly admired Georgio the ICU orderly, danced me from the wheelchair onto the commode. Meena cooked my favorite lemon chicken, stuffed cabbage and beets, and threw them in the blender. One of our neighbors, J.B., was on call to help Seth carry me upstairs at night and down in the morning. J.B. was a rebellious young man at this stage, with a magnificent purple mohawk of great height and stiffness. He came regularly that weekend, bringing a crew of friends who carried me gently with hands interlocked to make a solid seat, my arms around their spiked heads.

My only sorrow that weekend was the much anticipated reunion with our dog Lucy. She greeted me enthusiastically, but when I hugged her head, I felt steel wool rather than her golden retriever silkiness. It was dysaesthesia, a neurological abnormality that painfully heightened my sense of touch. I was more than disappointed. My fantasy of the roomful of furry puppies had sustained me through so many nightmare hours, but now my own furry puppy was like a wire brush. But it didn't faze Lucy. She was pathologically solicitous of me. She would not leave me for a second, as if some instinct let her know I was needful of love and protection.

All my senses were screwed up, my sense of humor most and best of all. I laughed at anything, and my family laughed with me. We laughed when I dropped and spilled things. We laughed that I sounded like a drunk with marbles in my mouth. My first night home, I fell out of bed with a great crash that woke Naomi, who rushed in to save me and found Michael rolling on the floor with me, laughing too hard to help me up.

We laughed in part for our own protection. Did we sometimes laugh too loud to mask the "tragedy" of my illness? I don't think so. Our family had always been intense and, let's admit it, earnest. We'd done too little laughing per lived minute. We were always planning for the future: the next film, the weekend, college. All of a sudden the future was gone, too fragile to imagine, and there was just the moment. It was hilarious. Such naches.

INSTITUT DE RÉADAPTATION DE MONTRÉAL

❧ Autumn ❧

Journal: October 30, 1987

Day 1 at the Institut was lonely and strange. Everyone around me is in wheelchairs and I resent being in one, and fear it may be permanent, as it seems to be for most of the others. But on the other hand, being around all these sad, broken people may serve as motivation to work hard and GET OUT OF HERE!

Who wrote these journals? When is she going to wise up? I want to add footnotes to make sure every reader understands that when I wrote the words: "sad, broken people" three months after my stroke, it was because I believed wheelchairs meant powerlessness. I wanted only to return to normal, to be "the old Bonnie" again. I couldn't conceive of coming to terms with being disabled, let alone a

world where differences could be accepted and accommo-
dated as a right, not a burden. I want to place warning
signs with flashing lights around all the frightened stereo-
types of disabled people that litter my journal pages:
Danger—Bad Attitude.

But I have to let the old Bonnie speak for herself. I
can't demand that she know what took me so long to learn.
And sometimes she still lurks underneath. The journals don't
lie even though they sometimes reveal my ignorance and
fear. Even though they are shot through with silences, events
unconsciously ignored and avoided as I tried to write my
life into a happy ending.

~

I arrived at my new home by ambulance. Michael wheeled
me down the hall to the admissions desk, past necking teenagers with cerebral palsy, amputees, quadriplegic ex-bikers
in black leather jackets. I had never seen so many wheelchairs. Michael was giddy, flying, telling me over and over
how happy he was. I could see why he liked it: the JGH was
old and dark, with hospital-beige walls. Here at the Institut
everything was open and light. Bright walls were plastered
with Don't Drink and Drive posters (*L'alcool c'est Volant*).
But I couldn't match Michael's enthusiasm. The warm colors seemed false, the poster warnings too late for many of
the residents.

After a series of admissions formalities, I was interviewed
by a psychiatric consultant called in to assess my panic attacks. He talked to me for over an hour, questioning me

about my childhood and unresolved feelings about my father. I eventually asked to leave, pleading exhaustion. He reluctantly agreed that I could continue psychotherapy with Michele Devroede, as I wished, instead of becoming his patient. Actually, we weren't called "patients" at the Institut, nor were we "residents" or "clients." In French we were *bénéficiaires*, which sounded awfully like "charity cases" to me.

Finally Michael took me up to my new room and my new roommate. Paulette was not happy to see me; I could only guess that she'd had the room to herself for a few days before I was admitted, and liked it. She didn't respond to any of our introductory chatter and curiosity. I didn't realize she could hardly speak. I didn't yet know that she'd been in the hospital for over a year, that she never had visitors, that her youngest child had been killed in the car accident that permanently injured her own brain, that her husband had subsequently abandoned her and their two young sons, who were now living with her elderly mother. All I knew was that when she decided to say something, it came out as an unintelligible drawl—I couldn't even tell that it was French. Did I sound like that too?

When she left for supper in the cafeteria, she went from fierce scowls to extravagant, sky-lighting smiles, which scared me just as much. How could an adult human being have become so like a child? She's brain-damaged, I told myself. Like me.

I was crying for the first time since I had the stroke. Maybe I had been afraid to cry before, scared that once I started I'd never stop. I didn't even know I was crying until I tasted the salt on my lips. I couldn't feel the tears running down my face. Michael wiped my cheek. I yelled at him, asking why he was so happy when I was still in a wheel-chair, still in an institution. He said, "I did all my crying before, when it looked like you might die. Now all I see is your progress."

After I was thoroughly comforted, Michael left for din-ner. Mine was brought to my room by a six-foot nurse's aide in a red dustmop wig, rosy cheeks, striped socks, and a white apron: Jimmy Deakin as Raggedy Ann, on his way to the *bénéficiaires'* Halloween party. Jimmy explained that since I was new, I would not have to go down to the cafete-ria but could eat in my room for a few days. My special puréed dinner had not been ordered yet, so I was to eat regular food—steak and *frites*. Whoopie! After Jimmy left, I wolfed it down, choking on the gristly meat. I would cough up the culprit and regurgitate it whole. Then I would chew it more slowly for the juices, and spit out the bolus. It was thoroughly disgusting, but I was alone so why not? I was enjoying myself until I suddenly got scared that the meat would get irretrievably lodged in my throat, and I would choke and die alone in my room, like someone in a grim tabloid article. How could Michael have left me alone in this place? Luckily, Naomi, Meena, and Anne Usher ar-rived before that dire fate overtook me, and I was suddenly as up as I had been down before. Anne reported that the halls were full of people in costumes, and persuaded me to go down to the cafeteria with her for the Halloween party.

The party seemed to be run entirely by the *bénéficiaires*. The room was loud and joyous and thick with cigarette smoke, sending my one unparalyzed vocal chord into spasms. I had never seen such an array of disabilities—the neurological ward at the JGH was mostly older patients with strokes and Parkinson's—and here were all these weird people dressed up even more weird for Halloween! There were paralyzed princesses, peg-leg pirates, beggars, and monsters of all description. There was a beautiful Cleopatra borne in on her litter by three or four dashing paraplegics. She won the prize for best costume. I learned the next day that she was always horizontal. Still later I learned that she used to play flute.

Jimmy Deakin put me to bed that night in what became a nighttime ritual. He brought me milk and cookies and chatted about his kids and mine while I ate. He helped me go to the bathroom and brush my teeth, then positioned me for the night. He knew just how to arrange the pillows for ultimate comfort and support. I didn't miss the JGH at all.

Over the next week I was seen and assessed by all the departments at the Institut. The neuropsychology tests were endless and sometimes humiliating: memory, problem-solving, pattern-finding, picture-drawing, deductive reasoning, abstract conceptualization, what's-wrong-with-this-picture? I kept feeling as if I was doing terribly, that I had lost my ability to think logically, to recall, to discern. The worst tests were the ones where you were supposed to figure out sequencing patterns of numbers, at which I had never been terrific. I see now that according to the consultation report,

I didn't do badly, though they didn't tell me then. I had a nagging feeling for a long time that yes, I was functional, good enough for them, but I had lost a great deal of my intellectual acuity. I wasn't sure I was "all there." I didn't know what might be missing. My thinking was slow. I reversed syllables, fractured idioms. "The ball's in your park," I'd say. "People who live in glass houses shouldn't throw up." I often couldn't find the name for something and would have to describe its attributes: "That thing with the long handle you use for sweeping the floor."

This new relationship to language wasn't entirely negative; I became sensitive to hidden meanings, the literal ones, buried in familiarity. It was fun making these new discoveries. Dis-cover. Re-member. In-valid. As in the work of Mary Daly, the feminist theologian, words fell apart, revealing their insides. But these gains could not be measured on their tests. Only the losses showed.

> **Michael:** Some of the effects you experienced—difficulty concentrating, inability to deal with more than one thing at a time, trouble with choices and decisions, scrambling words—are in a sense "typical" of people with stroke. Part of stroke is extreme fatigue; your terrible illness, your struggle to stay alive and recover, made you completely exhausted. The same is true of personality changes: you had extreme, exaggerated responses; you were inappropriately accepting or frighteningly demanding; you loved or hated. There were abrupt mood swings; you laughed too loud or cried without provocation, were often irritable and totally disinhibited. These characteristics all increased with fatigue.

Journal: November 6, 1987

My funk of the last few days was relieved by several factors:

1) One of the doctors assured me that most people get depressed at this stage of rehab—after all the life-and-death drama is over and the long slog to recovery lies ahead.

2) I woke up this morning to blood on the plastic sheets—my first period since the stroke! I had been looking forward to menopause and the end of my menstrual cycles, but now I celebrate the return of normalcy—even PMS!

3) Joe Carlton came to visit. He repeated his absolute faith that I will keep improving, and reminded me that we have a tennis date. Seeing Joe again made me realize: I HAVEN'T HAD A SINGLE PANIC ATTACK SINCE I GOT TO THE INSTITUT! When I last saw him, they still ruled my life, and now I take their absence for granted.

So I'm feeling joyous again, though TIRED in the extreme. What a yo-yo I am! The smallest thing can either send me flying, or shoot me down. The OT intern helped me lease a lightweight wheelchair yesterday and when they asked if we wanted to buy instead, she said: "No, it's temporary!"

Later that week, as I pushed my way to yet another test, I spotted André, a man who had crewed for a day on *Mile Zero*, with one of the Institut administrators. I'd known André for years. Michael had helped his partner with the delivery of their baby. I greeted him spontaneously. To my dismay, he did not recognize me. I had to introduce myself by name.

André recovered from his embarrassment with a quick

brainstorm. He was here as Location Manager for a made-for-Quebec-TV-movie to be shot next week at the Institut. Could I show the actor (heart-throb Michel Coté) something about using a wheelchair? The story line was about what happens to his love affair (with the talented Marie Tifo) after a car accident disables him. No, I'm sorry, I couldn't. Well, would I come down to the shoot as an extra? It would be fun for me, just like old times to be on the set.

Hadn't he noticed that I was no longer Bonnie Klein? Did he want the whole world to see me as part of a freak show? I could hardly hold myself in a sitting position in the wheelchair. My head hung crookedly. The right side of my face drooped down: mouth, chin, eyebrows. My eyes were usually closed. I looked, acted and felt like a Stroke Victim, the kind of person you try not to stare at. And that was in a still position, doing nothing. As soon as I added any movement, my strangeness was magnified. If I got excited, confused, or stressed, I would cough uncontrollably, spewing spittle. My legs bounced around of their own volition as if they had nothing to do with me. I hadn't yet learned how to stop their mortifying movement with pressure from my hands. Lesley Levy urged me to remember that I was still the same person I'd always been, but I couldn't bring myself to believe her.

How could I expose what I had become to a camera?

But André was persistent and sent messages to my room about the call schedule for the shoot. I avoided it most of the week, worn down by the endless batteries of tests. In the end, my curiosity won out. I went downstairs to occupational therapy ("*ergo*" in Institut-French) on the final day of the shoot. They were filming an emotional scene with the actor relearning to drive in the simulated *ergo* half-car. The filmmakers greeted me with what felt like sincere delight. Then I was directed for the action: the camera would start with a close-up of me, and pull back as I wheeled up a ramp to reveal the star crying in the funny car. It crossed my mind that this cameo appearance was like a Hollywood in-joke: name-that-crip. But I gritted my teeth and did my bit—several takes while the camera operator timed his zoom to my slow-motion ascent.

$\sim$

After my week of tests, real life finally began. I was given an *horaire* or schedule, like at school. Every day I had an hour of *ergo*, an hour of *ortho* (speech therapy), plus an hour of speech lab (supervised by a computer which graphed my voice as I spoke, feeding it back to me while I struggled to make the sound look right). Practical details like eating, going to the bathroom, or wheeling down the long corridors to my next appointment took up most my time in between formal sessions. It wasn't summer camp, it was boot camp. Luckily, I would have a furlough at home every weekend.

Ergo was first thing after breakfast. The *ergo* intern taught me how to dress and bathe myself, all in carefully thought-out stages. I learned to put on my bra by hooking it in front and turning it around, to pull up my pants while lying on the bed, to put on my sneakers and socks. Laces were beyond me. Thank God for Velcro!

My roommate Paulette could shower herself. I couldn't imagine the strength and courage it would take to transfer from the wheelchair to the plastic bench in the tub, especially when wet and slippery. The *ergo* intern taught me the steps involved and the safeguards, till I was ready to try by myself with a nurse's aide standing by *au cas où* (just in case). I had to line up my wheelchair exactly parallel to the plastic bench, lock the brake, remove one of the detachable arms, and transfer from the chair to the bath-bench by wriggling my bum slowly over the "chasm" from chair to bench.

Once there, I had to adjust the water temperature, starting always with cold for safety and remembering that I couldn't feel enough to keep from burning myself. Only then could I begin soaping and shampooing, pushing a lever to switch to the handheld shower hose to rinse. I invariably soaked the toilet paper roll across the tiled room. Toweling myself dry was another problem. I couldn't tell which was moving, me or the towel. I would as likely move myself off the seat.

My toileting traumas continued at the IRM, where I had graduated to using the regular bathroom (with help) during the day. It was particularly stressful in the morning. They routinely gave me a stool softener, Colace, because sedentary people tend to get constipated. But sometimes my problem was the opposite. My morning bowel movement was stimulated by breakfast tea. It came with a sudden cramp. The cafeteria was on the ground level and my room (and bathroom) was on the second floor. I had to wheel to the elevator and then wait for it to arrive and be loaded—

only four wheelchairs at a time. By the time I got to my floor I was desperate. I would yell from the elevator door that I needed an aide for the bathroom and pray that one—preferably female—got there before I shit my pants. By this time I was well enough to feel humiliated by men helping me onto the toilet, which increased my motivation to manage it by myself.

The maneuver to the toilet was tricky—especially with flaccid sphincter muscles. There was a floor-to-ceiling pole, like a fireman's pole, in front of the toilet. I'd position and brake the chair, reach for the pole and pull myself up while the aide pulled down my pants—there was no way to get my pants down myself, as I was clinging to the pole with both hands. Then I would pivot around to sit on the toilet.

The aide would usually leave me to do my business in private. When I was finished, I would buzz, and wait on the toilet until rescued. There was a ward of quads—that's what they called it—down the hall whose needs were much greater than mine, so I sometimes ended up sitting there for quite a while.

Eventually the *ergo* intern taught me how to wiggle my pants off with one hand, an inch at a time, while holding onto the pole with the other. I wore nothing but elasticized waists for years—buttons and zippers were out of the question.

At night the bathroom was inaccessible. Our wheelchairs were parked in the hall after 10 p.m. so the staff could get to us without tripping over them in the dark, but it meant I was stranded. My mattress had a plastic sheet over it for the inevitable bedwetting.

~

My *ortho* (short for orthophoniste or speech therapist), Miriam, was an orthodox Jewish woman (an ortho *ortho?*) with a wig, recently married and now pregnant, who had a sweet smile and childlike voice. Was she patronizing me? Or is this an occupational hazard when you work with people with language problems?

Miriam took me under her ample wing. We worked in English, which was a welcome respite in my French-speaking day, but she was tough. I had the feeling she thought I had lost more than anyone else acknowledged. She noted each mangled word and fed it back until I got it right. She was a stickler about my posture, always nudging me to sit up straight, stop slumping, don't let my mouth hang open. I thought she just didn't want me to look sloppy; she didn't tell me that how I sat affected my breathing, which in turn affected my vocal production.

Miriam was strict about "homework" which she wrote out in large, clear print. A patient patient, I was conscientious about my practice, and proud. There were strengthening exercises for my tongue: trying to touch the tip to the roof of my mouth and around the insides of my lips and cheeks. I had to do these in front of a mirror, which forced me to see how grossly distorted my tongue had become. It was red-raw and quavery, so thick it was almost square, making speech and swallowing more awkward.

After *ortho* I was ready to collapse in my room. Alongside my bed was a wall-to-wall window overlooking a large field. It was the first time in four months that I could see the world, the weather, the changing of the seasons. The far end of the field had the autumn vestiges of a large vegetable garden: corn stalks, tomato vines, sunflowers. I later learned that this was a communal garden—not for the Institut community (and why not? but that's a question I would only ask myself years later)—but for the neighborhood, a tidy jumble of fifties-style duplexes.

I spent hours staring out the window, listening to Peter Gzowski, Bob Kerr, and Jurgen Gothe on the CBC. By my bed I kept my journal, my *Friends' Book of Healing,* and my precious radio and cassette player. And joy! I had a generous window ledge running the width of the room for all my treasures: audio cassettes, family photographs, books and magazines, asters from Irene Kupferszmidt, my humidifier. Children's art was taped to the clothes locker and, as always, Naomi's poem was by my bed.

Between my double vision and my eyes bouncing around, I had not been able to read for a long time. Now my eyes were calming down, and I tried reading newspapers and favorite magazines. Exhaustion made it impossible to concentrate; I could not keep an idea in my head from the beginning to the end of a single sentence. When I found myself rereading the same sentence more than three times, I knew it was time to wait for a more alert moment.

Over the next months and years, what I wanted to read most of all were accounts of people who had been where I was—and recovered. Michael and Lesley gave me Bernie Siegel's work, *Love, Medicine, & Miracles,* about patients'

role in their own healing. Other wise friends gave me books
by Oliver Sacks. *The Man Who Mistook His Wife for a
Hat*, which I had ignored for all the months it was on
bestseller lists, gave me the first intriguing clue that there
might be another way to look at "abnormality": as difference, uniqueness, or even gift. I devoured his books. *A Leg
to Stand On*, about Sacks' own story of temporary neurological disability, became part of my growing collection of
personal narratives of illness survived and transcended, what
author Nancy Mairs ironically calls "the literature of personal disaster." I read about Patricia Neal's recovery from
a stroke and relearning of language, Helen Keller, Norman
Cousins, May Sarton . . . After years of reading nothing
but earnest non-fiction, I attacked fat novels like Isabel
Allende's *House of the Spirits*, rediscovering the pleasure
of fiction.

Journal: November 10, 1987
Yesterday was frustrating—back to the Institut after a weekend
at home, to do the same boring *ortho* exercises and still no
physio. If rehab is going to take as long as people anticipate
then let's begin. I'm angry at being here, and feel less optimistic
than I was. No one will guarantee full recovery. When Michele
Devroede came for our session I was crying (again). I told her I
was just feeling sorry for myself. She encouraged me to go
ahead and feel sorry, it wasn't going to impede my progress.

I was eager to begin physio, which for me was the only
thing that counted; it meant learning how to walk. But for

the first few weeks I was told I wasn't ready. Considering I had made such "miraculous" and speedy progress in so many domains, including the leap from scribble to legible journal writing in a few days, I secretly believed that it would be the same way with walking. I would get up from the wheelchair, stagger for a few minutes, and walk off needing only a few corrections.

I was pleased when my *ortho*, Miriam, told me that my assigned physio, Michel Danakas, was one of the best in the Institut. But when I finally was allowed to begin physio, Michel merely dropped by from time to time to check up on me; my body was in the hands of a nervous young intern who needed even more reassurance than I did. I had no confidence that she knew what she was doing. And after the exalted Michel Danakas told me I should stop my acupuncture sessions with Bernard, I didn't have much faith in him either. "If you do so many therapies at once, how can we tell which one is working?" he asked. "I don't give a damn which one works," I muttered to myself. "I just want to get better." It seemed like typical professional chauvinism. Bernard said no one thing was responsible for my progress; we were a team, all of us, including me.

The intern spent weeks "assessing" me: measuring every minute angle of movement; testing and timing my reactions to hot and cold, sharp and dull. The testing seemed irritatingly pointless to me, but it was also tiring, and I needed many rest stops when I would just lie still on the mattress, which seemed irritatingly pointless to the intern. At the very end of our time she'd stretch my arms and legs, and do some passive range-of-motion exercises. After a few weeks of this and a few awkward weekends in bed at home, I asked her if she could stretch my groin so it would be possible to have intercourse. She pretended not to hear me. No one ever talked to me about sex: no physio, no doctor, no OT, no psychologist. Michael and I figured it out ourselves.

But for all its frustrations, going to physio meant going to the gym—the centerpiece, the place of honor, the nerve-center of the Institut. It was a huge room with a wall of wide windows running its length and lacquered, blond wood floors scattered with glossy red and blue vinyl-covered mats. The therapists wore bright t-shirts, Hawaiian shorts, psychedelic sneakers and sweats. To my surprise, I was excited by the visual spectacle. The sunlight was fractured by window blinds creating dancing patterns of light on the figures within. And the figures themselves were dancing. *Bénéficiaires* and therapists became partners in the most original of *pas de deux*. Winch-transfers were breathtaking lifts, and leg stretches were transformed into sensual intimacies. The practical techniques of physiotherapy created endless configurations of body parts, one arm stretching to reach the other's hand, a leg on the other's shoulder.

That was the view from my filmmaker's eye, but my other eye flinched from this display. I hated seeing the droolers at the gym (though I also drooled). There was a young couple who always seemed to be slobbering. I wanted to yell at them, "Control yourselves, you're grown-ups." They flailed their limbs around with no control, contorted their mouths to utter stretched words I couldn't discern, and hooted their laughter, or was it grief? Everyone at the gym was always joking and raucous. The patients pulled tricks on the therapists and the therapists teased the patients and everyone laughed their heads off. Most of it was grade-school humor about colostomy bags and impotence. I thought it was sick: what do these people have to laugh about? (In truth I envied their camaraderie.)

Evenings everyone gathered in the lounge at the end of the corridor to watch television and smoke. I remember wheeling in there one evening early on and feeling repulsed by the slapstick comedy they were blasting in French. My CBC-classism was offended. I wasn't even into the hockey games, which blur those class lines for other people, mostly men. I asked myself, why should I socialize with these people? We have nothing in common. This is only a passing phase for me: I'm going to be healthy and "normal" again soon.

I certainly didn't think of myself as a snob. "Some of my best friends were working class." But they were the upwardly mobile exceptions. We knew each other within a middle-class context—the NFB or Herzl—where middle-class attitudes were the unacknowledged rule. I had never been in the minority before. I wondered if maybe working-class people had a higher percentage of accidents. But one friend laughed when I suggested that. "This is a more accurate representation of Canadian society," she said. "It's your life that's been distorted."

∼

I tried the lounge again on the day that the former Quebec premier and nationalist hero René Lévesque was buried. All of Quebec was glued to the television. I watched this moment of history in a room full of broken mourners, feeling my Otherness more than ever.

Michael was surprised by my uncharacteristic unfriendliness. But I wasn't interested in befriending any of these people, it was too threatening. Among my own friends, I was different and special now. Here I wasn't at all special, just another cripple among cripples, a little luckier than some and unluckier than others. My doctor-husband was unknown except as a visitor like other visitors. I was stripped of all the roles which defined me to myself and gave me status. Nobody knew of my films; nobody spoke my language.

I told myself I had no extra energy to spend on anything but rehab work. I sat alone in the cafeteria so I wouldn't have to talk and people wouldn't see me gag, choke, spit out, and spill. I used a paper bib, which an orderly tied around my neck. It was always repulsive after I ate. The smoke made my choking worse. Smoking was tolerated even in the non-smoking areas. The rationale for such lenience in a health institution, full of respiratory disorders, was that "handicapped people have so few pleasures." All the staff, from the chief administrator on down, were smokers, and the legislation was cheerfully ignored.

My room was my haven. It was the only place besides the gym and the therapy rooms where there was no smoking allowed. But Paulette was there too, hiding out like me, from what I never knew. She had one tape only: Bob

Marley's *Confrontation*. I was excited because Seth played it at home. But soon I felt if I heard "Chant Down Babylon" one more time, I'd go crazy. If it wasn't Bob Marley, it was the French Top 40. I would ask her to please turn the radio off when she left the room, but she'd be gone for hours and leave it blaring. For me to turn it off meant a transfer from the bed to the wheelchair and inching my way around the narrow aisle to her bedside table. I did it once or twice and she was furious that I had touched something of hers. She had so little: a bouquet of plastic flowers, a little Christmas crèche, and her radio. She was right to be protective, because one time, in my fumbling, I knocked over her crèche and it shattered. When she came back to the room and saw it, she threw the pieces at me and didn't speak to me for weeks.

Between the tension in my room and choking from the smoke in the cafeteria, it was hard to find a place to visit with friends. They came bearing homemade lunches and tasty take-out dinners to fatten me up, as I had lost about thirty pounds and was desperately skinny. I looked forward to the food, but I was far too tired for conversation. When the dictatorial Michel Danakas sent word that I should limit my visitors to one a night instead of cramming them in over lunch and during my afternoon break, I was relieved rather than angry at his presumption. Weekends became the focus of my social life.

Michael came for me the minute my Friday afternoon speech lab was over, and brought me back to the Institut just before curfew Sunday night. The second weekend he devised a plan to bring me back early Monday morning before the 8 a.m. staff meeting at Herzl that began his week. I thought it was bad for him to begin his week after a night of sleep interrupted by my restlessness, but he thought it was a brilliant idea, and from then on I was three nights home, four nights at the Institut.

Friday nights I was too tired for anything but Meena's Shabbat dinner and an early bed. Starting Saturday morning, however, our home became the kind of open house I'd always dreamed of, but had never made time for. Saturday night potluck dinners were a weekly event. Michael and Naomi took over the host role I had previously monopolized. I learned—not without difficulty—to be less perfectionist when they didn't do it *exactly* as I would. Naomi would serve chips to Rabbi Ron's little kids in a breakable family heirloom. Michael had a habit of putting out everything as it arrived, including desserts, which might be followed by cream of broccoli soup. I was shocked to discover that we now had a microwave oven, smuggled from New Jersey by Annie and Philip. We'd never had one before because Rosalie Bertell, from *Speaking Our Peace,* said they emitted cancer-causing radiation. When I objected, Michael told me that since he and Naomi were doing the cooking, they would do it their way.

Seth continued to come home every weekend. I was worried that he couldn't be developing any kind of social life at university, but he was unambivalent about coming. One of our weekend rituals was showing off my new accomplishments to Seth. I wouldn't tell him so I could see if he noticed "Mom's new trick." He was always wildly impressed.

Through his eyes I could see my real progress, too often masked behind the everyday grind of exercises at the Institut.

I knew I looked strange. I was desperate not to be an embarrassment, especially to Naomi. I remembered the easy humiliation of my own teenage years. But "normal" was an act I had forgotten. I cursed liberally and discussed my toilet needs; I was what the physicians called "disinhibited." Once I was lying on the sofa when Naomi came in with her current boyfriend. I heard my laughter, loud, deep, and rhythmic, at some dumb joke I had made. All the insults of childhood pointed their fingers at me. Grinning idiot. Retard. Spazz. I had never used those words about anyone else; why was I now using them against myself? Was that how Naomi and her boyfriend saw me? Was that who I was? I asked Naomi about it later and she reassured me that she thought I was very funny, and that she was nothing but proud of her mom.

I hadn't seen my own mother for three months. Michael thought that seeing me in the hospital would only confuse and upset her. Naomi and Meena both visited her; I don't think Michael could handle it.

Now that I was out on weekends, a visit was possible. Her nursing home was inaccessible, so Seth and Michael brought her to our house. I was dreading her reaction to finding me in a wheelchair. Naomi helped me fix myself up so I looked as well as possible. But when they brought her into the living room, she just smiled vaguely. All those weeks of worrying about her reaction and she had none. She barely knew me. I didn't feel relief but terrible loneliness. I had thought I'd accepted the Alzheimer's before but this was the moment of truth. It was as if I had no mother. When she left I couldn't stop crying. Seth tried to comfort me, saying, "Perhaps it's a blessing that she's not aware of what you've been going through." To which Michael sadly replied, "Such naches."

Michael lost no time inventing adaptations for life at home. One of my biggest problems was getting someone's attention from room-to-room with my still thin voice. Michael's solution was a walkie-talkie, the children's toy variety. It worked fine, as long as it was turned on, and in the same room as other people. As a fail-safe he bought a green plastic whistle, also from the toy department, which he hung from a turquoise necklace. It was shrill and effective when I remembered to wear it.

I used a rented commode, placed indiscreetly in a corner of the dining room, until I mastered the chair-to-toilet transfer. Then Michael installed a vast array of stainless-steel grab-bars, which medicalized the look of our old Victorian bathrooms. Even with the bars, I didn't have enough leg strength to get all the way up or down from the toilet, so we resurrected the big plastic raised toilet seat from the basement where it had lived since my mother moved to the nursing home.

Because the upstairs bathroom was down a long corridor, I needed a bedpan for the night. Everyone was so matter-of-fact about the commode and bedpan that I never felt humiliated. Michael put a rubber pad under the sheet; he never seemed put off by his incontinent partner. We delighted in the warmth of sharing a bed again.

Lucy and I were close friends, with all the time I spent exercising on the floor. She thought it was a delicious game. I was a sitting duck for her retriever tongue, and I incorporated her licks and smooches into my exercise routines, even though her hair in my mouth (like everything else) made me choke. My weekly comings and goings upset her, and she developed a phobia about suitcases. Whenever she saw a bag in our bedroom or stairs she would lie beside it moping, or follow me around the house, refusing to leave my side.

I had a daily physio routine at home. Michael was scared to let any time go by when I wasn't working. Every doctor who saw me, from Joe Carlton to Skip Peerless, warned that there was a "window of opportunity" for relearning before recovery became less and less possible, a limited time period when the nerves could find new pathways around the damaged areas, after which, progress would cease. Did I have a year? Two years? No one who explained this theory could be more precise.

There was yet another race against time. Michael drew me a graph with a gradual upward curve for recovery, and a downhill curve for the natural process of aging. I had to recover as much as I could before the lines intersected and recovery was overtaken and reversed. It made sense because my deficits were similar to those that come with natural aging, when reflexes slow, balance wavers, muscles weaken, tremors set in. This graphic information created enormous pressure. The window of opportunity was closing like a vice. My old age would be even less mobile, so I'd better get to the highest point from which to begin the downhill slide.

I ask myself in retrospect how much my fierce motivation was for Michael's sake. His graph was not a threat but a picture of his fears, drawn to urge me on in my recovery, which I translated into an image of the burden I might be on him in my old age. I had to get as well as I could for him. The obligation was self-imposed, but the race concept was truer to Michael's nature than mine.

~

I had another immediate priority. It was on an early November weekend that Sidonie brought over a videotape of her three-hour cut of *Mile Zero,* and my work on the film resumed. I watched it alone, in half-hour segments over several weekends, as I couldn't sit any longer than that. I was eager to begin, but there were moments when I questioned the wisdom of it. Was it too early in my recovery? Was I squandering energy on the film while the window of opportunity slowly closed? Should I be in *ergo* making potholders instead?

The first work session took place in our small living room, with Irene-the-co-producer, Sidonie-the-editor and me-the-director-with-a-stroke. In documentary film, this is where the interesting work begins. Since documentaries exist in the director's head, there is no script. Hopefully, you've captured the "reality" during the shoot; now the film begins to tell you what it's about and your work is to shape and heighten that meaning.

As we watched and talked I was not sure what I could

contribute. I didn't know how much mental ability I had lost. The neuropsychologist and the speech therapist at the Institut both led me to believe some loss was inevitable. I spoke very slowly and sometimes forgot what I was saying in mid-sentence. I hated when someone else finished what they thought I was going to say; it undermined what little confidence I had left. I couldn't cope with being asked two things at once, or even sipping water and watching the film at the same time. When Irene spoke too fast or worse, interrupted me, I got frustrated and angry, and lost my train of thought completely. Sidonie has the proverbial saint's patience, but Irene tends to be quick. I couldn't keep up. I felt loss of control.

During one particularly difficult session, the thought crossed my mind that maybe my work on *Mile Zero* wasn't real. Maybe Sidonie and Irene were humoring me—letting me think that I was contributing to the film because they thought it would help my healing. When I dared to ask Sidonie about it, she reassured me that she would never participate in such a charade—I was still the director, it was still my film.

Journal: November 20, 1987

I returned to the Institut exhausted from my wild weekend. I had worked two half-days on the film. I felt more confident than last week—I can work—slower than before, but perhaps better, more focused. When I work, I forget to take my Xanax.

Michel Danakas scolded me for wearing myself out on the film. He says my real work is at the Institut.

Xanax, a tranquilizer, and Ludiomil, an antidepressant, had originally been prescribed to help with panic attacks back in London, but I was still taking them. I'd always been cautious about any drug which affected the mind. I'd heard too many stories of tranquilizers being casually prescribed to women. Michael respected my fears but assured me that this was an appropriate use of those drugs. When I no longer needed them, my body would help me phase off.

For now, I was desperate. Desperate to avoid a return of the panics, or panicked because I was addicted, I couldn't say. I was prescribed Xanax every four hours. My heart palpitated for the last minutes before each dose. When visiting hours ended at 9 p.m., I started looking at my watch and listening for the meds wagon in the hall. When Jimmy came around with the juice and cookies, I'd ask him how far down the hall the nurse was. She seemed to be dispensing meds later and later, sometimes she hadn't even begun. I couldn't wait another half hour. I pestered Jimmy to tell her I wanted to go to sleep early, so could she please bring my medications right now. I was hooked.

At home on weekends, I took responsibility for remembering my medication. There was little danger of forgetting. By now I usually recognized the signs: chest pains, shakiness, falling apart. Xanax time! When I became very involved with something, like working on *Mile Zero,* I might not notice that I had passed the four-hour interval. When I noticed, I panicked. Quick, the Xanax, quick! Any time I went out of the house, the little bottle was standard equipment. In fact, I had several little bottles, *au cas où.*

Journal: November 30, 1987

American Thanksgiving weekend. This has been my best
Thanksgiving ever, despite some ups and downs. In the afternoon, Annie and Philip were in the kitchen preparing the
turkey. I'd had my weekly deep muscle massage and was left
alone in the living room to rest on the massage table. After
awhile, I was stiff and uncomfortable and I called for help to get
down. No answer. My whistle was upstairs, as usual. I called
and called until I was hoarse and terrified. It seemed like hours.
When Philip finally came, my fear became anger: "Why did you
have the radio on when you knew I was all alone and you're
both hard of hearing?"

Philip felt terrible and I was immediately ashamed.

We had made up by the time the guests arrived: Isabel, Bernard, Sidonie, Terre, and soon after that, Joe Carlton and his
wife, Susan, whom I had never met before. I was sitting on the
couch and Terre was in my wheelchair, and Susan mistook her
for me. Terre strung her along for a few minutes, in our old
"Terre Klein and Bonnie Nash" routine. Everyone thought it was
hilarious, including Susan, but I was suddenly upset by it. I
didn't like seeing Terre in that chair. I didn't want anyone I
loved to be in a wheelchair. For Terre, it was just a place to sit,
but for me it's a hated symbol. I cling to the words of the *ergo*
intern who said it was only temporary, and to the Peerless prediction: if I'm not exactly standing, at least I can get up with
support to transfer from one chair to another.

After a few tears that no one but Michael noticed, my mood
swung again. Here I was, at home with family and friends, and
no nose tube. Thanksgiving!

I wanted to somehow consecrate this occasion, but I knew of no appropriate ritual. I couldn't look for the words in a book, or wait for someone else to say them. If it was going to happen, I would have to create it.

At my request, Michael tapped on a wineglass before dinner and everyone became silent. I spoke spontaneously, without much breath or volume, about the intimate connection between love, healing, and giving thanks. I became aware in the silence that I was speaking holy words—words the old Bonnie might have been embarrassed to speak. But I'm tougher now. If I can forthrightly discuss my bowel movements, I can certainly risk a little holiness in my own dining room.

❧ Interlude: Holy Shit! ❧

Journal: March 10, 1995
As a culture we are hung up about secretions and excretions, the stuff of our bodies. There's not even any casual, everyday language for them; the words are stiffly scientific, or baby talk, euphemisms, curses. This society is set up so that non-disabled people can pretty well pretend they never pee. But when I was sick, that's what my life was about. There were always secretions from my mouth. I coughed up great gobs and spit them into tissues.

I choke a lot too, then and now. Sometimes I have a choking fit in a restaurant. We often ignore it ourselves until people at neighboring tables start to panic, looking at Michael as if he's a murderer. "Not to worry. She does this all the time."

I no longer fill my sheets with diarrhea, but it sometimes happens that a piece of soiled toilet paper sticks to my bum and my still-numb senses are not aware of it. I used to go on my way, wondering where that lingering smell was coming from, examining the bottoms of my shoes for the culprit. Now I've learned to check, always check, after wiping myself. Then there's pee. Although I've regained control of my bladder under normal circumstances, I still wet my pants during choking spasms, or when I sneeze or laugh uproariously. For a while I hoped it was just temporary and took to carrying a change of underpants in my backpack. Finally I succumbed to those advertisements I'd always loathed and tried maxi-pads, which give me the promised security.

It took a long time and a lot of denial and humiliation to reach this point. Michael was not encouraging. It was a confusing switch, after the matter of fact warmth he showed during my days of total incontinence. When I wrote maxi-pads on the grocery list, he often either "forgot" to buy them or told me that I had "millions of boxes" around the house. He was slower than I to accept the fact that they were now a permanent part of my life. And he—this is hard to write—commented once or twice when the bathroom smelled of urine-soaked pads—I was saving the earth (again) by trying to recycle old bags that may have been full of holes. When I sensed his disgust, I felt disgusting. I eventually confronted Michael about his uncharacteristic squeamishness, and he's never since forgotten to add either maxi-pads or baggies to the grocery list.

"We demand the right to pee!" writes disability activist Joan Meister. Lack of accessible washrooms limits the lives of many disabled people. It's amazing how many public places will tell you that they're wheelchair accessible and it turns out their toilet is down a flight of stairs. Or the washroom is too narrow to fit a wheelchair. Or there's no grab-bar. Or the grab-bar is installed too high. I have a friend who drinks no liquids all day if she's planning to go out in the evening. I have other friends who just don't go out. Unholy details can determine where we live, work and go to school, not just whether we go to the occasional movie. It's not the shit that's profane, but the exclusion.

We don't have the luxury of politely ignoring our excrement. We have to think about it, talk about it, plan ahead, strategize, write petitions, lobby governments, chain ourselves to buildings, change the world, or else pee our pants.

❋ Winter ❋

I finally complained at my weekly medical exam that I wasn't getting adequate physio. The next day, as I was absorbed in my stretching exercises, Michel Danakas himself came bounding across the gym floor. He bounced on my mat with an exuberant "Bonjour Bonnie!" I flinched away in panic, burst into startled tears and hit him with my weak fist. Michel knelt beside me. "*Eh bien, qu'est ce qui arrive?* What's happening?" He put his arms around me and I soaked his t-shirt with tears and snot.

I started working with Michel every day. Like Iolanda before him, he was a cheerleader. "C'mon Bonnie, you can do it. *C'est beau, c'est ça,* that's it." He had noted my first fear-reaction and incorporated it into our sessions. He would throw me off-balance and we would end up rolling around and laughing on the mat. He would urge me to resist. "*Pousse! Pousse!* Push! Push!" he'd say, sounding like an overly enthusiastic childbirth coach. This was a "serious" exercise to develop specific muscle groups through resistance to pressure. But with Michel it was also playing.

I bounced from nervous anxiety to giddy laughter to desperate determination. Around the gym I was a known workaholic. Michel was always trying to get me to ease up. My friend Guy would roll by and tease "*Lâche pas,* Bonnie, *lâche pas.*" ("Don't slack off, don't let up.") I started each physio session on my own with stretching and strengthening exercises. Michel would keep an eye on me as I worked, and join me on the mat at a certain point. He would stretch me further, just beyond the point where I had imagined the limit, and then move on to various arcane exercises. I can see now that they were for developing reflexes, balance, trunk control: necessary precursors to walking. But back then I was still waiting for the moment when I would rise from my chair and walk away.

I could always look around the gym and see someone struggling with a skill that I had just mastered. I'd also see people who hadn't been at the Institut very long, doing much more than I could. Older stroke patients especially depressed me because they often went from severe paralysis to walking while I was still slithering on the mat. "He's eighty years old and using four-point canes already. What's wrong with me?" Michel would remind me of the difference between a brain-stem stroke and a hemispheric stroke, but in my heart I was comparing my progress to theirs and despairing. Occasionally I spent the whole session crying on the mat while Michel lay next to me, patting my arm.

I wasn't learning to walk. I was learning to use a wheelchair. It seemed like a waste of time to work so hard perfecting a skill that I would soon leave behind. But I had to admit, it was easier to get around. I stopped crashing into walls, and I even enjoyed the speed I could work up when I wasn't too fatigued. But whenever I rolled over a bump, I thought I was tipping backwards. I would freeze in the chair, eyes screwed shut, hands clenched, breath coming in small screams. Michel assured me the anti-tip wheels in the back would keep the chair from flipping over. "But it's the sensation of falling, not the reality that scares me," I would say.

I had lost trust in my body, in the ground beneath my feet. But maybe I'd always been a chicken. I wasn't raised to take physical risks. My parents sat shiva the first time I went skiing. Naomi never tires of telling how, after ten years of downhill skiing, I would get to the top of a chairlift and yell ahead to the attendant, "Please help me off; it's my first time." I didn't lie about many things, but this was life-and-death.

Michael had always encouraged me to face down my physical fears, and I had followed him up mountains, down rivers, and under oceans to justify his faith in me. I had also learned to listen to the wisdom of my own body. I liberated myself from downhill skiing in favor of cross-country, and chose yoga over squash.

Now Michael was encouraging me to face my fear of falling. "It's not the end of the world," he'd say. "Get Michel to teach you how to fall safely."

Michel did not agree. He was mortified when I fell. "No fall is a good thing," he'd say. "Our purpose is to keep you from falling." I was with him. I fell a lot, though never while learning to use a new piece of equipment. I would often lose my balance from a sudden turn, or misjudge the distance between two places, or throw my body on the floor in a brain-scrambled attempt to swing a door closed.

Michael had the bright idea to hire a private physio to work with me over the weekends. How could I rest for two whole days when the window of opportunity was steadily closing? Michael was not a natural rester: "No pain, no gain."

Michel was appalled. *"Lentement mais surement! Slowly but surely."* I was convinced. I told Michael—it was probably a direct quote from Michel—that healing takes place in the resting as much as in the working. He backed off then. He's a bad rester, but a good learner.

At last Michel said I was ready to work on the parallel bars. These were two handrails running the width of the gym, with a mirror at either end. I transferred from my chair by grabbing the bars and pulling myself up with the upper-body strength I was earning daily in the gym. What joy to be upright! I would take halting steps, grasping the rails for dear life. When I dared look up from my feet, the mirror showed me the difference between where I perceived my body to be and where it really was in space. I could correct my position, unlock my knees, untwist my pelvis, relax my shoulders, straighten my head. So much to remember. The scariest part came when I reached the end: I had to let go with one hand and (gasp) trust that I could stay upright while pivoting around till I could grab the opposite railing and switch hands for the return trip. I felt like a performer on the high-wire.

At first Michel stood beside me, helping to support my weight as I stumbled along holding the bars. Then, as my balance improved, I did it "in harness" with a wide leather belt around my waist and a strap for Michel to hold *au cas où*. I had often seen *bénéficiaires* in harness, leading their physios along the corridors or across the lobby. This was the last stage before "real" walking and the glamor of their independence made them seem less like leashed dogs. Soon I'll be off the bars and walking the halls, I told myself.

Finally Michel brought out the *marchette*, the same three-sided walking frame I had been learning to use at the JGH before my second stroke. We started by walking short distances in the gym. I was supposed to take a step, then lift the *marchette* and place it ahead of me for the next step. But what would happen to me during the time that the walker was off the ground? How was I supposed to stay up? What made them think I could do this?

Walking with the *marchette* was an enormous strain: supporting my weight, standing upright, shifting to lift one leg, remembering to bend at the knee, to step down with the heel first. A rote litany. "Look ahead at where you want to go," Michel would remind me. "Don't look at the floor."

But how else could I be sure the floor was still there, when I couldn't feel it beneath my feet?

It took many weeks, but I did it: three steps, five steps, halfway across the gym. Michel lavished praise on each nervous victory. "WOW!" he'd say, in about ten syllables. "WOOOOOW!"

Michel Danakas: I remember going back to the office, sitting down, completely drained. Working one hour with one person can be as tough as working with eight. But then there are seven other people waiting for their time. You were one of the tough ones like that. On a scale of ten, you were around nine. When someone says they want to walk by next month, then I say to myself, oh, oh, watch out. If their expectations are really high, then whatever I do won't be good enough because they don't progress fast enough for their dreams. I felt like I held you only by a small string, and some little thing might cut the string and you would give up.

Journal: December 10, 1987
Michael came to see me in physio but he didn't find me at first because he was looking at wheelchair level and I was up with the *marchette*!

I can walk the length of the gym now, using the *marchette*, and I jumped my leg weights from 1/2 lb to 1-1/2 lbs. This week I continued going to the bathroom alone in the daytime. I pulled up my pants with two hands! At night I still wet the green plasticized sheet and buzz for the night nurse when the cold wakes me.

Ergothérapie (occupational therapy in English) was like home economics for absolute beginners, with a functioning kitchen and mock-ups of bed, stairs, bathroom and the half-car that appeared in André's film. Everyone was assigned a partner, and we played games and did projects together. My partner was Denise, who lived across the hall from me. She was more sociable than Paulette; in fact, she never stopped talking. She was a full-time housewife from the suburbs: not my type, I once would have thought, but now we were friends. She'd had delicate spinal surgery to remove a malignant tumor and was praying it would not recur. Michael was not optimistic about her prognosis, but I reminded him that people had not been optimistic about mine.

The *ergo* lab with its large collection of children's games, could have been a place to play as adults (like physio down the hall). Instead, the therapists proceeded with humiliating seriousness. We worked at shuffleboard and ping-pong and navigated obstacle courses. We did pre-kindergarten puzzles with large wooden pieces, carnival games with clown-face targets, and uninspired paint-by-number crafts. Denise devoted herself to a pre-fabricated wooden nativity scene for Christmas, while I made potholders.

A high point came when Evelyne, our *ergothérapeute*, asked Denise and me if we would like to prepare a lunch, and invite our respective physiotherapists. It took something like two weeks to prepare this extravaganza, including planning, invitation-making, writing shopping lists, the wheelchair excursion to buy groceries at Steinberg's supermarket in the mall across the street, and finally cooking, setting the table, serving, and cleaning. If the purpose of the activity was to encourage us to resume our culinary activities, it convinced me that I could either cook or have a life.

Journal: December 13, 1987

Razelle is here for the weekend! She walked into the *ergo* lab yesterday, hugged me and cried: "She's moving!" She stayed for an hour and Denise and I showed off our prowess at bean bag toss. Tonight we ate at L'Impromptu, my first outing. I had a moment of self-consciousness wheeling to the bathroom, which passed. The bathroom was wheelchair accessible—with proper grab-bars!—in spite of the small size of the restaurant.

When we came home, it was just starting to snow, but I made it up the steps clinging to the rail and Michael's arm.

Winter looked beautiful until I tried to wheel in the snow. I could no longer roll myself down to the car when Michael arrived to pick me up, but had to wait for him to help me through the slush. An unshovelled walk was as impossible as a curb for my chair, and far too slippery to negotiate with the *marchette*. At home, there was no sidewalk from the driveway to the front door, just a path across the lawn. After the first big snowfall, Michael purchased a thirty-meter strip of indoor-outdoor and rolled out the red carpet for me. It got pretty filthy and forlorn after a Montreal winter, but it served its purpose.

Chanukah came early that year, shortly before the

Institut's two-week winter break when almost all the patients went home for the holidays. Seth was supposed to make it back for the first night's celebration. Unfortunately his train got stalled in the snow just outside of Montreal station and he ended up sitting in a tunnel for two hours before the tracks were cleared. On the second night Seth came to the Institut with Naomi and Michael and our Chanukah menorah to light candles with me. One of the Mitzvot of Chanukah is to put the lighted menorah, a symbol of the miracle, in a window so it can be seen by passersby. I saw it as a gesture of openness and pride about being Jewish in a predominantly non-Jewish culture. Besides, it is very beautiful to watch eight candles burning against the winter night. Do we transport this tradition to a shared room in a Catholic hospital? My husband and children did it without hesitation. We chanted the three blessings and even sang some Chanukah songs. To everyone's surprise, most of all my own, my usually discordant singing voice came out sweet and sure. What miracles a paralyzed vocal chord can accomplish.

The Herzl Chanukah party was on a weeknight, so I got an evening pass from the Institut. It was a chance for me to get dressed up and see people who'd been so important to me when I was at the JGH. For the last ten years, the party had been a potluck at our home, but this year it was at a gigantic Chinese restaurant that claimed to be wheelchair accessible. When we got there, we discovered that "accessible" meant that the waiters would be happy to carry me up the stairs. Michael was furious. I, on the other hand, thought it was a great adventure to be escorted on a freight elevator full of garbage through the bowels of the kitchen, and then carried up the remaining stairs by several strong family practice residents.

As it turns out, I didn't last long. I learned what was to become a pattern (and persists even now): the anticipation of such an event, and the kerfuffle around accessing it, plus the excitement of being in a crowd of people, exhausted me. I didn't even make it past the hors d'oeuvres, let alone the dancing. I couldn't wait to go "home" where Jimmy would tuck me into bed.

～

Two weeks of winter break at my real home was heaven. That was the holiday when I learned to dance. I don't remember how it started, whether it was another of Michael's bright ideas for therapy, or a spontaneous moment that just happened in the privacy of our living room. Maybe Michael noticed my unruly feet tapping to the Preservation Hall Jazz Band, trying to dance my body out of the wheelchair. At any rate, he quickly rolled back the carpet (my feet stuck to rugs), took my hand, and we jitterbugged to Louis Armstrong, Benny Goodman, Ike and Tina Turner. I usually had trouble shifting my weight from one foot to the other, but dancing somehow allowed me to bypass all that left-brain stuff. The beat went right from the music into my body and my feet were released. My movements were rigid and jerky and Michael had to loosen my knuckles when his arm became white from my deathly grip, but I was dancing. Lucy ran for cover. Naomi, who used to get annoyed by any physical expressions of emotion between Michael and me, got a big kick out of watching from the stairway. Once she even deigned to dance with me herself.

Terre Nash: During Christmas break you brought home the *marchette*. You used it all over the house. You would walk to the kitchen, sit down and rest a while, and then walk to the dining room. I said to you, "Remember the Peerless prediction: 'Standing by Thanksgiving, walking by Christmas.' And look at you now, it's true!" But you got mad. You had thought that walking by Christmas would mean really walking. Using the *marchette* didn't count.

Journal: January 4, 1988
The holidays went too fast. Monday morning was glum—back to boot camp after two weeks at home. Michael slept badly and cried when he brought me back to the Institut. Then he called at noon to remind me that we both get depressed on Monday mornings.

Paulette was discharged before the break and is now an outpatient, with physio three times a week, except so far she hasn't shown up. It seems strange, but I miss her. We maintained a tenuous peace for a while and then Michael managed, with many small courtesies, to win her over so that she sometimes even smiled. I cheered (and envied) her achievements as she conquered the four-point canes and then began walking by herself. In exchange, she kept the radio lower and even turned it off when she left the room. The real breakthrough was when her two small boys came to celebrate her birthday in their Sunday best. My admiration for her lovely children overcame her defense, and she expanded to a beaming grin. We had not bonded as survivors of brain injuries but we bonded as mothers. I hope she comes back for physio—Michel says most outpatients don't.

I'm wondering if I'll be ready to leave by the end of January as promised. Everyone I know who's left could walk on their own and I can hardly last for five minutes on the *marchette*, I'm shaky as hell on my new four-point canes, I can't walk *down* steps without a great deal of fear and support, and I still tire easily though less than before. Michel thinks another three weeks is a lot of time to improve, so I'm still aiming for it, though I'm trying to prepare for the possibility that it might be wise to wait longer. Progress at this point is much less dramatic and visible, so I have to fight the tendency to get discouraged.

My new roommate is twenty-five-year-old Martine, who had a car accident two and a half years ago. She spent four months in a coma, and has been hospitalized ever since. She seems positive and cheerful.

Martine had an indulgent mother and a doting fiancé named Stefan. The story was that she'd had another boyfriend with whom she was driving when she had the car accident that landed her in the hospital. She and Stefan became a number sometime afterwards. One night I recounted this to Michael. He pronounced the relationship "sick;" "pathological." Why? I wondered. Was it sick for an "able-bodied" man to love a brain-injured woman? And if so, what did it say about us?

I was afraid to ask such questions. Many people in the Institut were alone. Some were from far away, separated from their families by too many miles for regular visits. Others were simply abandoned. Most husbands leave their wives (90 percent according to one unsubstantiated statistic) and almost half of women leave disabled husbands. Even more shocking, many disabled children are deserted. I didn't want to think about it.

Journal: January 15, 1988

I had a bad experience in *ergo* this morning. An old patient of Evelyne's came by to say hello—he walks with one cane and is still unable to work after two years. I wonder what he does all day. Evelyne offered him as a hopeful model, saying he was like us when he began. All I could see was the cane and the limp, and I got suddenly depressed and tearful. When Evelyne asked why, I said I'd expected to go much further, in fact to play tennis this summer. Evelyne broke into uncontrollable laughter at the idea, it seemed so preposterous. I was devastated. She apologized later, though she said she'd be enormously surprised if I could ever run again. She allowed as how it might be helpful to hold onto an image, however unrealistic. She said she hoped she hadn't been too brutal in making me confront reality.

I spent the rest of the day in my room, without the energy to continue. Part of me refuses to believe her, refuses to give up. The other part says there will be no more heroics, no dramatic recovery, just days and weeks and months of hard work with no defined endpoint, no light at the end of the tunnel. What's the point? After the ecstasy of survival, what exactly have I survived for?

❧ Interlude: Talking Back ❧

Journal May 26, 1995

Who said revenge is sweet? They're right, it's delicious.

Well it wasn't exactly revenge, it was even better. I was invited to give the Keynote Address to the Annual Meeting of the Canadian Association of Occupational Therapists! The profession has decided to become "client-centered"—the jargon of the nineties—and are admitting they don't know exactly what that means. So they invited me—the ultimate mouthy client—to talk on their theme, "Partners in Practice."

What an opportunity to turn almost eight years' experience to good use! We in the disability rights movement say that we are the experts about disability, that we long to de-medicalize rehabilitation and take it into our own hands.

After congratulating their commitment to partnership, I innocently asked whether any of the 600 people in the room besides myself considered themselves disabled? As I suspected there were no hands. I pointed out the inherent power inequality in their hoped-for partnership, the unspoken barrier between helper and helpee, provider and consumer, have and have-not. How hard it must be to treat people with disabilities as equals if they don't have daily, ongoing contact as peers and colleagues.

I told them the Evelyne story. When I said I had expected to play tennis, there was a titter in the room. I acknowledged that it is laughable in retrospect, that Evelyne knew much more than I knew. She also knew that not being able to play tennis or even to walk wasn't the end of the world. She knew that there is life after disability. But I didn't know that as a person who had just become disabled. And she did not try to bridge that gap. I never trusted her after that, never bonded to her.

It's arrogant of anyone to impose limits on another person's healing. People with disabilities are always telling stories about "the doctor said I'd never do this or the therapist said I'd never do that." We've all defied odds and predictions. Why? I think the reason some people "succeed" more than others with similar conditions is a combination of factors: social and economic circumstances, motivation, and the support of family, friends and therapists.

I proposed that OTs consider themselves our *allies*—clinically and politically, that rehab professionals fight the handicaps that are imposed on us not by our impairments but by societal attitudes, and help us remove the barriers which restrict our movement in the world. No one ever prepared me to live as a disabled person in a world that is often hostile and excluding. I felt like I was the first person in the world to use a wheelchair.

If society doesn't have a place for us then we can't value ourselves. How can somebody have self-esteem when everything around them is telling them the opposite—that they're not worth the additional expense of a Braille version or a personal care attendant or American Sign Language, that these are frills affecting only a few people?

I no longer see independence in terms of how far I can walk, as I did in physio, but as control over my life, measured not by tasks I can do without help but by the quality of my life with the help that is needed. That's a more radical definition than the conventional one, and I think more interesting for therapists than teaching us to play checkers or even to walk, and probably closer to the reason most people become rehab professionals in the first place.

I think my speech touched a nerve—I even saw a few tears. Perhaps it's not naive to hope that "client-centered" will be more than the latest catch phrase, and perhaps someday a partnership of equals can be forged around our common strength and vulnerability.

OUTPATIENT

I left the Institut on Valentine's Day. After more than six months of living in institutions, I was ready. My last days were endless. I hated the unchanging routines, the cafeteria food, the bright posters on cold walls. I hated the sight of sweet Jimmy Deakin wheeling the juice and cookies down the hall at night. I was lonely. It was not my home.

On the other hand I was terrified of being discharged. I felt as if the rehab system was giving up on me. Rehabilitation from a stroke is often declared to be complete after six months, or maybe a year. In a strictly cost-benefit analysis, there were diminishing returns for the medical system as my progress plateaued. The high drama was over, and the rest was less interesting for the health professionals.

I don't remember if we had any sort of homecoming ceremony. When Michael grabbed the scissors and cut off the hospital bracelet, marking me a free and well woman, I would have liked to say the *Shehechiyanu,* a Jewish prayer of thanksgiving, which freely translated means: "Thank God we've lived to see this day!" But we probably just grinned.

Nothing was impossible now. We had handled the commode, the carrying up and down stairs, and now I was so much better. It was going to be easy. Meena was going to come full time, so I wouldn't be alone while Michael was at work and Naomi at her new English *cégep.* I would continue at the Institut as an outpatient, work on my film, see my friends, be a real wife and mother.

Everything would return to normal.

Journal: February 18, 1988
Suddenly I'm thinking of myself not as ill, but as a well person (with a temporary inconvenience). Is that the difference between hospital and home?

I love being here. It's better than ever, because now instead of constantly sniping at each other, Michael and Naomi are a team, looking out for each other, strategizing for my comfort. On nights when Michael is on call and Naomi has a date, she takes his beeper with her and if he gets called in, she races home so I don't have to be alone. I can just imagine her dancing in some funky club with a doctor's pager clipped to her jeans.

I'd never heard of a Jewish ceremony for leaving the hospital, but renewing tradition is what Reconstructionist Judaism is all about. I spoke to Rabbi Ron who responded with enthusiasm: we would create a special Shabbat service. He brought over stacks of material about healing he'd collected from both traditional and contemporary Jewish sources: Hannah Szenes, Mordecai Kaplan, the Psalms, an adapted mourner's kaddish.

Ron and I compiled a supplement for the Shabbat service, and called it "A Celebration of Life." Naomi agreed to include her "Dear Mummy" poem and Seth wrote on what he'd learned about me, his dad, and his sister as we lived this crisis. I added Marge Piercy, Judy Chicago, Lao Tsu: "A journey of a thousand miles begins with a single step."

We put an announcement in the synagogue bulletin, and invited a few friends from Herzl and the NFB. Seth, an old hand at estimating political crowd size, said there were 150 people there that Saturday morning, including people we hardly knew, who had been following the course of my illness through Rabbi Ron's weekly updates at Shabbat services. My stroke had become a community event, reminding people of the fragility of their own lives and dreams.

I sat in the front row, with Michael and the kids and Annie and Phil who drove up from New Jersey with a vanful of homemade goodies for the event. Our family was called up for the first Aliyah, the blessing before the weekly Torah reading. I had been sitting through the service worrying about how I would get up the two shallow steps to the *Bimah*. When the moment came, Michael and Naomi took my arms and I managed it without stumbling. Everyone was silent. We stood at the open Torah scroll, and together we chanted the ancient sweet melody. Ron led the congregation in the *Shehechiyanu*.

Next came the *D'var Torah,* the Jewish equivalent of a sermon. Today it was not Rabbi Ron but Michael Klein who gave the *D'var.* It was the first time Michael, who had not had a Bar Mitzvah ceremony, ever spoke in synagogue. His *D'var* was a thank-you in the form of personal stories about the many ways people had helped us. He couldn't resist telling the story of Rabbi Ron coming to visit me at the JGH when I was unable to roll over. "Can I do anything to help?" Ron had asked. "Rub my ass!" I replied in my breathy, disinhibited new voice.

In the synagogue, when Ron asked if I wanted to say a few words, my heart was too full to speak.

Journal: February 23, 1988
I'm so tired of being tired. Every little activity is big. Like taking a shower. You shower before doing something, right? You shower before breakfast, or before you get dressed and go somewhere. But no, for me a shower requires going back to bed afterwards to recuperate. I nap throughout the day and still need to go to sleep by 7 p.m. every night.

It's the tiny things that get to me. I can't carry. It's only when you can't that you realize how much you need to. When I use the wheelchair, I can carry things on my lap, but now that I'm up with the *marchette* around the house, I don't have any free hands. We tried to saddle Lucy with a carry-pack but the old dog didn't tolerate this new trick. Michael suggested I use a knapsack, but it throws my balance off. Even carrying a towel around my neck is too much for my tenuous *marchette* skills. Pockets work, or holding things with my teeth, or dropping things down from the stairwell (except it breaks the backs of books). But I can't put a cup of tea in my pocket or throw it down stairs.

Spontaneity is a luxury. I have to plan ahead to remember everything I need, so I don't have to blow that stupid whistle for Meena to come help me. "Please bring me the phone, bring me my box of tissue." I try to ask nicely, but I feel so demanding, so . . . colonial. What is this white lady doing, blowing a whistle as if Meena were some dog?

Three days a week I went to the Institut for physio, *ergo* and *ortho*. Just getting ready to go was a big deal. I was much too shaky to use public transit by myself, and besides it was totally inaccessible. Montreal had never heard of lift-equipped public buses, and the Metro stations all had narrow escalators or steps. No one had prepared me for the world of Transport Adapté, the parallel transit system for people with disabilities. To qualify, I discovered, I needed a medical certificate saying I was "permanently disabled." I hated that piece of paper. It was a lie. I was getting better.

Transport Adapté had a few buses and special cars for people with electric wheelchairs, but for people like me, with folding manual chairs, they contracted out to private cab companies whose drivers were resentful of the extra time we took. I got the feeling that everyone at Transport Adapté was overworked, exploited, and angry. To book a ride, I had to call several days in advance, give them the exact address I was coming from and going to, and the exact times I wanted to be picked up and returned. I had to be ready at the door ten minutes before the reserved time, but they might not get there until twenty minutes after. Or they might be much later. Or my booking might have been lost. You were not allowed to call and check until after the allowable twenty minutes' lateness. The line was always busy. If you weren't waiting at the door when they arrived, they would leave. If I was at the Institut, where the phone was an absurdly long walk from the front door, to call or not to call was a big dilemma. If the driver showed up while I was en route to the phone or waiting on hold, then I'd miss the ride. Such is the drama of parallel transport. It was much easier to stay at home and, except for my outpatient appointments, that's mostly what I did.

The Institut was not set up for outpatients. They had a full roster of inpatients whose needs were urgent. We were a sideline, fit into the cracks of their regular program. When I'd been a "real" patient, I lay down in my room after lunch every day before I went to lab or gym. Now I ended up alone in a staff lounge feeling like a trespasser, eating my bag lunch and napping on the plastic sofa. By the end of the day I would be shaking with exhaustion, ready to go home and collapse if only the Transport Adapté would come.

On days when I wasn't at the Institut, I would practice walking on four-point canes. Meena would help me with my coat and boots, leash up Lucy, and off we'd go. I'd count my progress by house numbers and landmarks: one driveway down, then two, then all the way to the fire hydrant. I was so precariously upright that it seemed a wind or a passing car could knock me over. The slant of the side-walk felt like a steep ridge on which I was balancing.

For longer jaunts, Meena would push me in the wheel-chair. She took me shopping on Rue Sherbrooke, which was just around the corner. This was the neighborhood where I had lived for years, where I had frequented the old greystone shops without ever really noticing the steep granite step at each doorway.

Meena Williams: I know you didn't feel too pleasant some-times, always needing help. I don't blame you. It's hard to be in someone else's hands like that. Often you were ner-vous. It was good when Michael put that Mickey Mouse bell on your wheelchair, because you could ring it when you thought you might bump into someone. You had some control. But any unexpected noise, or a car that suddenly appeared would upset you. "Wait, wait, that guy's pulling out!" You had to depend on my eyes, my hands. And you felt every bump in the road. Sometimes you'd say, "Why didn't you steer around that?" But that's just the way the roads are. Especially in the snow. It was hard. This climate was not meant for wheelchairs.

When I became steady enough on four-point canes, I would carry them across my lap in the chair, and with much courage and Meena's help, I would ascend the few steps for a haircut at the local beauty parlor. This was the same place where I'd had my hair cut for years, rushing in at 5 p.m. after a day of work. Now a hair appointment was a major activity, only to be undertaken on a good day, followed by an afternoon in bed. I felt awkward; everyone stared at me, distracted from their chitchat and *Chatelaine Magazine*. As my hair was cut, I studied my face in the mirror. Had I changed? I was thinner, paler, but still recognizably me. I looked normal, even pretty. But then I stuck out my tongue and there was the Truth—thick and distorted, like a slab of raw liver—a monster tongue in a woman's mouth.

By this time a ramp had been installed at my mother's nursing home, so I went to visit her twice a week. But no matter how often I went, I always felt guilty for not going more. The first time, my mother got agitated as soon as she saw me. "Are you wondering why Bonnie's in a wheelchair?" Michael asked. She nodded, crying. Michael took her hand. "Bonnie was sick but she's better now," he explained, and that was the end of it. She always responded to Michael. I don't know if it was a faint echo of their old relationship, or just his deep male voice that she warmed to (as I had to Rick's). He could win a smile from her even on days when all I got was a blank stare.

I hated seeing my mother in that place. I hated the combination of love, pity, and recognition that rose in me each time I entered her tiny room. I had been there. I too had tried desperately to talk, only to be misunderstood or ignored. I too had been tied into my wheelchair and pushed from place to place. I too had waited in a bed of excrement for an orderly to come. "The difference is that you're getting better. And she can only get worse," Michael said. It was a cruel difference.

Journal: March 2, 1988

My doctor at the Institut said my main obstacles now were proprioception (not knowing where my body is in space) and coordination, problems that aren't easily addressed by therapy. He feels I will still make progress over the next months, though slower, and that we won't know till next autumn to what extent I am "functional."

I came home depressed.

When Michael first suggested we go to the Caribbean for a swimming holiday, it seemed impossible. Our idea of a vacation has always been camping in some out of the way place with strenuous hikes and unusual bathroom facilities. We looked down our noses at tourist traps that promised all the comforts of home. Why not just stay home then? But Michael was sure we could find both accessibility and adventure. We ended up booking a one-week package at a resort hotel in Guadeloupe.

At the airport everyone ignored me, asking Michael whether "she" could walk onto the plane, or if "she" needed the narrow Washington chair to board. My body got numb from sitting so long in the cramped airplane seat, but the narrow bathrooms turned out to be perfect; I could balance using the close walls and grab bars. I wondered how people who couldn't get out of their wheelchairs managed to go to the toilet.

I remember the hot wind on my face as we deplaned, the smell of ocean and flowers. I wanted to throw off my shoes and run barefoot on the beach. Instead, I sat on the hotel bed and cried. I didn't even know how I would get down to the water. It was too far in the walker and the chair couldn't wheel on sand. My body couldn't tolerate the heat any more than it could the cold in Montreal. Michael cried with me that first morning and then we made love in the bland resort room. I decided this was going to be a good vacation after all.

Journal: March 21, 1988

This is a vacation of small adventures that are more exciting than all the mountains we once climbed. We found an accessible beach not far from the hotel where I can walk right into the ocean with the *marchette*. Michael has been using all his old swim-teacher tricks to help me in the hotel pool. It's scary and hilarious all at once. I can't kick. I tried and tried, holding onto Michael's waist at the shallow end, but my feet won't move in any orderly fashion. I was holding on so tightly that I pulled his swimming trunks down. We laughed so hard I almost drowned. None of the other guests seemed to find it funny at all.

The other guests were mostly European tourists with bronzed muscles and designer swimwear. They would congregate on the beach or in the dining room, striking up flirtations and friendships. Michael and I sat alone. No one asked our names. No one said hello if we passed in the courtyard. They averted their eyes and tried not to brush up against me. My body was pale and emaciated, my muscles still slack from months of paralysis. I felt like I was polluting their paradise. I was their worst nightmare; a reminder of the mortality of their gym-toned flesh.

Journal: March 24, 1988
Today we were crazy! Today I went snorkeling. I think I agreed to try it out of a silly determination to act as if I could do anything. And apart from not being able to kick, not having enough breath to clear the snorkel tube, and having to be lifted in and out of the boat, it was great.

Everything I've always loved about snorkeling was still there: the kaleidoscope light, the day-glo fish. The water allows me to love my body and to trust it. I can't walk on land, but I can walk in the accommodating water. My almost constant pain eases with no gravity to pull me down. When I'm swimming, my movements are fluid, smooth. I feel free and strong. And I bring that confidence to ground when I emerge.

On our last day, we rented a jeep and drove across the island to an isolated area of rocky beaches. We found a flat spot overlooking the ocean and Michael wheeled me across the rock to where I could see the sunset. I asked him to leave me there for a while. He was a little puzzled but quite willing to go off and play mountain goat. I listened as his footsteps faded and then there was nothing but the soft sound of the waves. I watched the clouds redden. A heron flapped by. It was the first time in eight months that I had been alone.

Journal: April 2, 1988
My post-vacation reentry was at a new level of wellness. I went to the Institut without the wheelchair—only four-point canes!

Wednesday afternoon I worked on *Mile Zero* at the NFB. Being

there was a bit overwhelming. I couldn't sleep the night before
or for two nights after. I snuck into the building with Sidonie
signaling when the corridors were clear so I could avoid
gawkers. We had a fine work session and I realized once again
how much I like making films. My earlier insecurity is gone
now—I know I'm still good at it. I love persisting until it's just
right—even when it exhausts me.

At that point, we had *Mile Zero* work sessions at home
once or twice a week, and in between Sidonie called with
questions and progress reports. The film was starting to
take shape. It opened with close-ups of individual teenagers talking about their fears for the future. What emerged
was not their despair but their passionate love of life. I
cried every time we replayed it. The joy of living, the fragility of the planet: these abstractions were fierce and
immediate to me. Life was sweet and full and precious in a
way I had never known before.

By June the final edit was nearly complete and I took
time off to go to California with Michael. Our trip was
first planned as a week of visiting family; my big chance to
"meet" my new sister-in-law Lyn, whose voice and gentle
massages I remembered through the haze of my second
stroke. But now I had another serendipitous motivation.
While I was still at the Institut, a friend had sent me an
article about Emilie Conrad Da'oud, a dancer in L.A. who
was reported to work "miracles" with severely paralyzed
people. More recently, I'd received a letter from Susan Griffin, a feminist poet and philosopher, whom I'd filmed for

Not a Love Story. Susan had become profoundly ill with
what was finally diagnosed as Chronic Fatigue Immune
Dysfunction Syndrome, and was greatly helped by Emilie
Conrad Da'oud. Well, it was clear that I was receiving a
message in stereo about this Emilie. I wrote and asked if
she would meet me when we came to L.A. She had no workshops scheduled for that time, but she agreed to see me
privately for a very modest fee.

I didn't know what to expect. Emilie sounded so "New
Agey" in the article I'd read, talking about cellular knowledge and micro-movements and alternatives to the central
nervous system. This was not the sort of thing I would do
in my right mind, but then I hadn't been in my right mind
since last August. Our approach to stroke treatment had
been to try anything and everything; we called it the "no
stone unturned" method.

Emilie was no stone. She was a bit less exotic than her
photographs, and she spoke New Age with a very familiar
Long Island accent, but she was also darkly, dancerly beautiful, and exuded a passionate confidence. I liked her right
away.

The work started flat on the floor of our tiny motel
room, in silence. We concentrated on my breath. She asked
me to pay attention to any natural movement that occurred,
even a twinge in a finger or a jerk in my thigh, and to exag-
gerate it and follow it through. In a short amount of time,
I was moving my limbs in unaccustomed ways, swaying
and writhing in all directions in movements which Emilie
called "primal" because they imitate the evolution of the

species and each individual. There were no formal directions, just the natural movement of my body, directed from
the inside out. There was no right or wrong, not even a
better or worse. I was self-conscious at first. I wasn't used
to this formlessness. In physio, I told my body what it should
do; here I followed its impulses. When I relaxed into the
experience, I discovered my body wanted to do many of
the same movements I was struggling with in physio: the
reaches, the bridging, the balancing. I felt my body wanting to stretch itself, to push and test itself, by its own volition.
But unlike physio, the movements were smooth and var-
ied, no sharp angles but big curves in many dimensions.

"You're a dancer," Emilie said. How outrageous! It was
wild, sensuous and pleasureful. I felt totally alive.

In the next session Emilie added words, or rather sounds,
because their meanings were beside the point: JACQUES,
JACQUES, SATCHADANANDA (or was it CHICH-
INITZA?) Making these sounds caused my body to move
in strange ways. I became aware that all the parts were
connected; my speaking, my breathing and my movement—
which had been fragmented into *ortho, ergo* and
physio—were all related through my central nervous system! It seems so obvious now, but back then, I had lost all
sense of my body's integrity.

I'd invited Michael to this session at Emilie's home, not
sure how he would respond. His first, knee-jerk (read: medical) reaction to "someone like" Emilie would normally be
skeptical. He was not too hung up on credentials but he
was suspicious of claims of miracle cures, and made corny

jokes about "ass-holistic therapy." But as usual, he surprised me. Emilie, for her part, was warm and respectful of Michael, not a knee-jerk doctor-hater. I think she appreciated validation from a socially sanctioned expert.

Emilie started by showing us some videos about her work. Watching them, I was struck by the utter sexiness of her body moving to its own inner direction. I was amazed, and envious, at the suppleness of her torso, how she could move each individual rib. She laughed at my awe and taught me what she called a tidal movement that undulated through my body like a soft wave. "Movement isn't something we *do*," she said, "it's something we *are*." Later that night, I had my first orgasm since my stroke.

The brief weekend with Emilie restored my confidence in my body and my feminist respect for its wisdom, which I had lost in the passive helplessness taught by my months of hospital and rehabilitation. I was a dancer too! I could play as well as work with my body; I could have fun, pleasure, beautiful music. I could take control of my healing: no therapist knew my body as well as I did.

Journal: June 2, 1988

I feel as if I've begun an entirely new chapter in my rehabilitation, one which I'll be writing myself. I'm a little nervous about returning to the Institut as an outpatient. How can I integrate these seemingly contradictory approaches, one from the inside out and the other from the outside in? How can I choose what's more important: my gait or my dancing cells? Do I have to choose? What would Michel Danakas think if I told him about wriggling formlessly and aimlessly on the floor instead of doing ten repetitions of the genuflection on my right leg with control?

For the time being, I'll try to lead a double life.

Journal: June 3, 1988

First day back at the Institut, I was struck by how many of the same *bénéficiaires* were still there, though I was only gone two and a half weeks. It seemed like so much more.

In physio I practiced with ordinary canes. They feel so spindly and thin—how can they support me? It was tiring, but nothing like the first time with the walker or the four-point canes. I can do this! I was so thrilled I cried, and so did Michel.

But Evelyne, despite her pleasant welcome is de-motivatingly negative. She said that Denise will probably walk without canes, whereas I—if I'm lucky—might get down to one cane. No, I said angrily, I will do without them too. Who gave her the right to dismiss my dreams? Does she think that's her job—to stamp out "false hope?" What a difference, after Emilie's repeated encouragement that I will recover completely. I'm not going back to ot—why should I?

Journal: June 10, 1988

We got a letter this morning from Skip Peerless. He was astounded by the snorkeling pictures Michael sent. And he said he thinks I will still be recovering twelve to eighteen months from now! That's good news, because lately I've had trouble imagining how I will go from walking as I do now—with fatiguing instability and dependence on canes—to walking unaided. If the time frame for the transition is stretched, then it appears

more feasible. As the kids in *Mile Zero* say, you've got to believe
change is possible before you can make it happen.

Journal: June 11, 1988
"In the face of uncertainty, there is nothing wrong with hope."—
C. Carl Simonton

Journal: June 17, 1988
Michael turned fifty today—a reminder of that race against
time. Last night I dreamt I was at the Montreal Film Festival, on
a scaffold high up outside a tall building, delivering some urgent message. I woke up and took a few steps without canes.
Michael was ecstatic, but when I got to the Institut and showed
Michel, he said it was "not functional walking" and probably
bad for my body because I was so tense and rigid.

In July, Miriam had her baby and went on maternity
leave. My new therapist was Judith Blumberger, the head
of *orthothérapie*. We had nodded to each other in the hallways for months, but never spoken. She seemed nice enough,
but *ortho*, with its endless tongue exercises and rote recita-
tions, was one of the most tedious hours of my day.

Judith Blumberger: When we first started, you were still
the Perfect Patient—doing what you were told and never
asking questions. You had these word lists, twenty-five or
thirty monosyllabic words. You'd probably been doing the
same ones for months—ploughing through, from beginning
to end, every word on the list. The first thing that struck
me was that twenty-five words was too much. I told you to
pick a few of them. You just sat there and stared at me.

"What do you mean?" you asked. "Which ones should I pick?"

"Pick any ones you like," I said.

"But which ones?" you said.

I ended up choosing them because you couldn't. Then I tried to get you to say which ones were hard. You didn't know. You had been taught to say this list, but no one had taught you to pay attention to how it felt. You left that session with six words. I told you to start by *visualizing* yourself saying them well, rather than just sitting down and rattling them off.

I think you liked the visualizing thing, because at our second session you told me about Emilie and California. I got the impression that this wasn't something you talked about at the Institut.

At that same session, you mentioned that you had a lot of pain in your neck. I asked you to move your jaw and your tongue; sure enough, your range of movement was quite restricted. So I thought, "Well, she has neck pains and limited movement, she likes visualization, and she's been to California for therapy with a dancer. Maybe she won't think I'm too outrageous to propose Feldenkrais."

Feldenkrais is an approach to movement that focuses on inner awareness, visualization, and intention. What we did was to forget about speech exercises and work on the very basic systems. We followed your breath right down your spine to your pelvis. By doing subtle exercises for your whole body, you changed your voice, because speech involves your whole body.

You showed immediate gain. You were breathing better, your posture was better, and of course you were vocalizing better.

Judith used the word "elegance." She didn't treat my body like an awkward enemy I had to fight into submission. She didn't scold my thick tongue. A weight lifted from my chest. I breathed deeper, stood taller, walked like a dancer on my flimsy new canes.

Journal: August 8, 1988

This past weekend was the one-year anniversary of the "insult," as one doctor called it. I was thinking in bed how happy I am. People often remark how awful this year must have been, and in fact it was. But my overwhelming emotion is how exciting each day is, how interesting and wondrous the human body. I want to live it and pass through it, to go forward, not around. I don't begrudge the time; there's nothing else I'd rather be doing. Activities yield such immediate results, the feedback is so direct and positive, once your time frame is adjusted to the millimeters of progress. This is not to say I don't have moments of extreme frustration and impatience, perhaps more lately as I'm closer to "normal" and can perceive how far I've yet to go. Memory is both a joy and a torment. I can so easily imagine myself as the mobile person I was. A glimpse of a woman playing tennis, a photo of me swimming in a Vermont quarry, triggers instant tears. But even in the midst of a hurricane of grief, I know it will pass.

We spent the weekend in the country with Muriel Duckworth, exactly one year after our missed Hiroshima Day date. It was a perfect celebration. I felt overlapping emotions of extreme sadness—seeing familiar places and friends with whom I swam and danced, just a year ago—and extreme joy.

I even played tennis, holding onto the net with one hand with my wheelchair parked beside me, *au cas où*. It wasn't the same game that first taught me to enjoy my body—I missed the sweat, the swearing, the adrenaline of competition, the glee of winning. But my first hit was thrilling—I had no idea if I was anywhere near the ball till I heard that grand sound of connecting—Wow! I have more fun with the limited things I can do than I ever did before.

In the evenings back at home, Michael, Naomi and I started going to a local outdoor pool where I added swimming to my exercise regime, increasing the number of laps I could do daily. I did barre exercises in the water, stretching my calves and thighs. Michael sometimes stretched me, which was fun but embarrassing, as I stood with my foot on his shoulder, making involuntary noises as my muscles cramped and released. (What is that man doing to her?) Best of all—though I only did it on overcast days when the pool wasn't too crowded—was dancing. I transferred what I had learned on dry land with Emilie to the water where, released from gravity, my movements became liquid. I moved free-form, without strokes, sinking and surfacing, rolling and spreading my arms. I tried not to care what it looked like because it felt so good.

After swimming we would saunter home, Naomi pushing my chair, watching the sunset and the summer night come in. I loved those walks together, but Naomi fretted about the inevitable storms to come. "I can't imagine going through another winter where you can hardly even get outside. You should go away somewhere warm and not come back till spring," she said. I thought it was a brilliant idea, but Michael brought me abruptly back to reality. "What are you talking about?" he said. "I'd have to quit my job! Nobody can take a three-month vacation."

"I'll just have to learn to walk then," I said.

~

Why did I decide I had to go to the Degas mega-exhibit in Ottawa? And why did I decide to go cold turkey off my Xanax the day before?

Even though I don't like mega-shows, I do like Degas. The National Gallery had just opened and I was interested to see the new building. But it was also this itching worry about being left behind. It was as if everyone in the world was going to see this show and I didn't want to miss out just because I couldn't walk.

Seth offered to take me, which was the best reason to go. He and Michael had been on a canoe-camping trip the weekend before, and it hurt that I couldn't go with them. I wanted my own special time with Seth. I wanted to show my son I still had spunk and spirit.

This was one of those hyped-up art events where you have to make reservations and go at a set time. We were booked for 1:15 p.m., and Ottawa was a two-hour drive. If we left at 10 a.m., we'd have plenty of time. But of course I didn't manage to get myself together until 10:30 a.m., and then we had trouble finding parking. By the time Seth pushed me to the museum, we were late and I hadn't had any lunch.

I've always been irritable when hungry, but like everything since the stroke, it had become extreme. First would come the headaches, then the shakes, weakness, and confusion. It was one of those things that I needed to plan ahead to avoid, because once I was in that state, I couldn't figure out what to do about it.

Seth asked me what I wanted to do—lunch or the exhibit—a big mistake. Another post-stroke symptom is difficulty with decision-making. When I'm calm, well-fed and unpressured, choosing between two options is difficult. When I'm stressed out and hungry, it becomes a major crisis. I fell apart. I knew I couldn't miss the exhibit, because that's why we were in Ottawa. And I couldn't skip lunch, because I was already in a hunger panic, and it would only get worse.

The foyer was crowded and noisy. Down at wheelchair height I felt lost and claustrophobic. I had cramps and chest constrictions from the Xanax withdrawal. A museum guard was standing nearby, taking tickets and giving directions. I pulled on his pantleg to get his attention. I tried to ask him if we could still get in to see the show if we went to the cafeteria first, but I was in too much of a state to ask clearly. I stuttered and babbled, then broke down and cried.

Poor Seth. Here he was, a young man out in public with a mother crying about her lunch. Luckily, the guard seemed perfectly used to such goings-on and once he managed to figure out what I was sobbing about, he gave us his word he would let us in however late we were. Seth rushed me to the cafeteria, applied food, and the storm left as suddenly as it had arrived. All I remember about the exhibit is that I loved it. It gave me a great new insight into Degas' work, which I have now, of course, entirely forgotten.

Journal: October 20, 1988
En route to London, Ontario, with a video copy of *Mile Zero*—completed last week—in my suitcase. I'm going for a follow-up exam and a pilgrimage: to say thank you, here's the human being who was hardly present the last time around, and to flush out memories so I can put them behind me. My memories of London come in vivid waves of smell and sound, but few visuals. I want to see what the hospital looks like, and Peerless and Rick. I remember their voices well.

First stop: Mickey and Linda's, where we'll be staying for the next two days. I couldn't believe I'd never been in their house before—Mickey-and-Linda stories are so much a part of our London mythology.

Next stop: the Magnetic Resonance Imaging Unit—over a year since my last MRI. Last time I was on a respirator. I remember the horrible knocking sound, how claustrophobic it was, and how long I had to stay still. This time it was a piece of cake. I saw myself in the chrome of the machine as I was strapped to the table, eyes bright (and made up) "alert and smiling." Afterwards, Michael rushed out to see the pictures while I got dressed. He said he was relieved. Interpretation from Peerless tomorrow.

Journal: October 21, 1988
I heard Peerless' voice in the hall and recognized it. He was younger than I remembered—a low-key man in his fifties. After

the now familiar neurological test, I asked him for another "prediction" of my progress. He said he never imagined I'd be so far by now—so much for predictions. Unlike some neuroscientists, he doesn't think the healing is finished in a year with the rest relearning. He believes structural reconstitution of my nervous system is still happening. That was music to my ears!

I still have what appears on the MRI as a small black hole in my head—a fluid-filled space where the malformation had been—but it's apparently not a concern.

We went from Peerless' office to the ICU. I had told Michael that I remembered no one but Rick and Mary, but I was amazed at how many people recognized me (with a double take). They were excited to see me; they said their patients rarely return voluntarily to the scene of their nightmares. Memories came flooding back—the sound of the respirator, the "Blue Chair," the cry of "x-ray," the RT (respiratory therapist) whom I associated with ET.

The first thing Rick said to me was "I can't believe I've never heard your voice."

"This isn't my original voice," I said. "It's the sexy voice I always wished I had."

I wanted to tell him how much his care had meant to me: the cheery monologues; the effort to always tell me what was going on so I wouldn't be panicked; the positiveness of my "sexual" interest that told me I was alive. But everyone else was crowding around and I didn't get the chance to talk to him further.

Eventually, the excitement did me in and Michael took me back to the house where I napped before the Big Event: the "world premiere" of *Mile Zero*, played on video in Linda and Mickey's living room, and attended by Rick, Peerless, Adrian

and several other members of "my" hospital team. Irene and
Sidonie sent a telegram of congratulations and Linda produced
bottles of champagne.

I was a little nervous, watching everyone watch *Mile Zero*.
These were the people who had kept me alive to make this film.
I wanted them to like it. I wanted them to laugh in the right
places. I wanted to make them proud.

And I think they were. They laughed and listened and
clapped loudly at the end. For me, this was the real premiere.

When I returned to Montreal, plans for official premieres
in Halifax, Toronto, Montreal, and Vancouver were already
in gear. My friend Gerry Rogers was hired to coordinate
and publicize these events. They were all timed to happen
close together, to give a national feeling about launching
the film. At least one of the SAGE tour-members would go to
every premiere to do media interviews and answer questions after the screening. All four of them plus Irene, Sidonie,
and I would attend in Toronto and Montreal.

I think it was someone from the NFB marketing department who first suggested that I do media interviews. They
said that because the tour itself had received a lot of cover-
age, the press would regard the film as "old news." Besides,
the Cold War had inconveniently ended while we were fin-
ishing the film. They said we needed a new angle or *Mile
Zero* would get no publicity. My mid-film stroke would be
the perfect hook to grab media attention.

I was appalled. But Gerry took me aside and advised
me to consider it seriously. Several reporters had already

refused interviews, saying they had "done" the SAGE kids. Without an extra push, *Mile Zero* would die a quiet death and disappear into the NFB archives. Gerry insisted that talking about the film and my stroke didn't have to be exploitative. She reminded me of all the times Sidonie and I had sat around the Institut, musing on the parallels between healing, peace, and filmmaking. She quoted me back to myself: "When I'm overwhelmed with how far I have to go, I think about high school kids deciding to stop nuclear war." "Rehab is like filmmaking—you have to try things and risk falling on your face."

I told her that her memory was too damn good, and I promised to think about it. But all I could think of was the long list of reasons not to do it:

—My energy is still limited.

—My voice is still weak.

—I don't want to choke for five minutes on live radio.

—I don't want to distract from the film or steal attention from the kids.

—I don't want people to feel sorry for me, to think this is another sob story.

—I don't want people to say it's a good film because it was made by a cripple.

—I don't want other filmmakers to be jealous.

Jealous? Who could be jealous of a stroke? But I could hear the voices in my mind: "That Bonnie Klein. She even manages to get mileage out of being sick. She uses her stroke to get attention and promote her career."

I couldn't do it. The answer was no.

Gérald Godin changed my mind.

Godin was a popular poet, and a Member of the Quebec National Assembly. He had been the Minister of Culture for the first Parti Québecois government under René Lévesque. I didn't know him personally, but I had once filmed his partner, Pauline Julien, a passionate singer-songwriter.

Dorothy Hénaut was working on a film featuring Julien and Godin, called *A Song for Quebec,* and she asked Godin to come meet me.

He was a wiry, fervent man. The effects of a brain tumor, discovered and removed a year before, were evident in his slow speech and halting gait. Like me he made disinhibited jokes and laughed too loudly. He had a wicked sense of humor, both in person and in his poetry:

—What! You don't remember my phone number?
—Listen, *mon vieux,* you know
they removed a tumor from my brain
the size of a tangerine
well,
your phone number was in it

Although Godin was a politician, and certainly not supposed to have a hole in his head, he decided not to give up his seat in the National Assembly. He continued to speak and vote and represent his downtown Mercier district, and in the next election he received an even stronger majority than before.

He urged me to be public about my stroke. Being visible as a brain-injured person is a good thing, he said, because it breaks the great taboo attached to brain damage. He said it's important for people who are afraid of us to actually see us, but it's even more important for us to see ourselves. It's important that we get over the shame. He made me laugh, both at my extravagant new peculiarities, and at the people who turned away, embarrassed, or presumed to judge me for them.

I thought, OK, if Gérald Godin can address the National Assembly, I can face a few reporters. He had given me this challenge, and it wasn't to be ignored.

I was supposed to arrive in Toronto a few days early so I would be able to rest up between the press interviews and the launch. Unfortunately, Michael couldn't come until the day of the launch, but before I could panic, Naomi offered to go with me.

Gerry had booked us into a downtown high-rise hotel. The "handicapped suite" she had reserved was on the lowest floor, but that turned out to be the seventh, as the first six were taken up by ballrooms and convention halls. Newspaper reports of disabled people burned alive in nursing home fires filled my mind, but there was nothing I could do but cope with my fear, hope for the best, and thank God Naomi was with me.

Journal: November 25, 1988
Yesterday was hectic but fun. Naomi and I met Judy Steed from the *Globe and Mail* at 10 a.m., and talked through lunch at the Queen Mother restaurant. She'd already seen a preview copy of

Mile Zero and interviewed Alison and Seth, so I felt comfortable talking to her about the details of my stroke. I can't wait to see what she writes.

When Naomi said she was thinking of becoming a journalist, Judy invited her to come to the *Globe and Mail* the next day. She also encouraged *me* to write a book about the stroke. She advised me to start by making lots of tapes, interviewing Michael, our children, friends, doctors, etc. Then someone could transcribe the whole thing, plus my journals. But the next stage—selecting, shaping, editing—I don't want to face by myself.

I wrote my speech, and rewrote it, and rewrote it. Michael arrived, and I kept him and Naomi up half the night listening to revisions. I had spoken before film audiences dozens of times, but this was different.

When the moment actually came, I was ready. First Irene spoke about the process of making the film together; then Michael helped me up a makeshift ramp to the stage. It was my decision to have the premiere at this inaccessible venue. The fully accessible educational institution that was our other option seemed boring compared to the glamorous and elevator-less Bloor Cinema with its splashy marquee and washrooms one floor up. I decided I'd be fine as long as I drank nothing all afternoon. I didn't think about other wheelchair users who might come, and (of course) there were none.

Journal: November 29, 1988
The Toronto opening is over. There was a standing ovation before I spoke, which made it hard to get the words out. I hadn't

thought they would stand and clap like that.

The film took on other dimensions with a responsive audience cheering and laughing at unexpected places. The discussion period was full of excitement, with the SAGE kids fielding the questions. Seth was at his relaxed best, full of impassioned analysis and humor. "If we were to take all the money devoted to nuclear weapons, we could find a cure for acne."

After all these months of worrying, I now see that the film *was* my rehabilitation—occupational therapy as it was no doubt meant to be. *Mile Zero* was real, useful work: it required all my previous skills and experience, plus many new adaptations; it connected me to the larger world outside my body; it forced me to "come out" and be seen in public; and it brought me validation as a productive person. I have regained a sense of my self.

☙ Interlude: Rosalie Sorrels ❧

Journal: July 17, 1993

The Vancouver Folk Music Festival is my idea of heaven: mountains, ocean, sky; a wide expanse of green liberally sprinkled with wheelchairs and guide dogs; accessible toilets; ASL interpretation; and music from around the world. Seth drops by the patch of shade where I have parked myself and Gladys, full of the workshop he just attended. He is particularly moved by an American folk singer named Rosalie Sorrels. The Festival Program notes that she had a brain aneurysm and "almost had her last gig in the choir of angels."

"You have to interview her for your radio show," Seth says.

Rosalie Sorrels looks weathered by a hard life; a down-to-earth folk musician of bars and back alleys, not coffee house cappuccinos. She walks only a bit tentatively. We trade stories, stunned at how similar our experiences were, and how different.

Rosalie Sorrels: Suddenly, one day, walking into my cabin in Idaho, I felt as if someone had hit me in the back of the head with an axe. There was no warning. I said, "Holy shit!"—those would have been my last words if I had died. I went down like a stone. My daughter tells me I got right back up and said, "There's something wrong with my head, you have to get me to town." She said, "I'll call an ambulance." I said, "I'll kill you if you call an ambulance; we can't afford an ambulance."

I live in the United States, you understand, where you don't have health insurance unless you're rich. So my daughter got some people who live nearby and they took me to a doc-in-the-box. He said, "She's having a migraine. Give her an aspirin and take her home." Now if you give someone an aspirin when they're having a hemorrhage it makes their blood go thinner, which could have killed me.

My daughter took me to another doctor and he said that's not a migraine—she needs a CAT scan. And I jumped out of this dying stupor, shot right up and said, "How much will that cost?"

They found an aneurysm—and a surgeon. He was very good. He shaved every lick of my hair off, opened up my head and fixed me—there's one chance to do it; take a tiny little clip and pinch that flaw shut, and then somehow make it so it will repair itself. I have no idea why I lived through all that but I'm terribly pleased.

The bill was very large, and the people I owed it to were very unpleasant. Friends across the country had benefit concerts and raised about half of it. Then the hospital put me with a collection agency and sued me. The only way you can live through that is to not own anything. Luckily for me, I own my dog and my guitar and that's it. So they settled for $800 instead of the many thousands they were suing me for, because that seemed to be my net worth at the time.

When I got out of that hospital I couldn't walk. No one from the hospital looked at me again because I didn't have any money. I was very mad. I got a walker and I taught myself to walk. I went out every day and walked as far as I could and then I came back, which was twice as far as I could go! And pretty soon I'd feel like I was strong and I'd put the walker down and I would fall. And I'd pull myself back up and start again.

I'm sixty years old, you know, these parts don't last forever. But I can't afford to get sick. In the States, whenever you talk about there ought to be health insurance, people start saying well who's going to pay for it? I know that's not the case in many other places. Once a person is alive in the world, it's the responsibility of everybody to help see that they get through it. I mean we're all a family after all; the world is a family and you take care of your family. You don't ask who's going to pay for it; you all get busy and figure it out.

I was moved by this tough woman's vision of the human family. And struck by the contrast in the medical care we received. In Canada, I was hospitalized for over six months and in formal rehabilitation for another year and a half. My only personal costs were for all my long-distance phone calls and $46 for a few days of TV in my room. The real cost to Canada's universal health care system (which we are not even told)—for those months of intensive care, the air ambulances, the surgery, the rehabilitation institute, the outpatient care—was more than $150,000 Canadian, around $120,000 U.S. (at that time). We were able to supplement the basic coverage with private medical insurance through Michael's employment. This covered certain equipment, Gladys, for instance, and medically recognized therapies like massage.

Neither Canadian health care nor private insurance covered any of the complementary therapies—like acupuncture, cranial massage, chiropractic, or nutritional supplements—not to mention Feldenkrais or Alexander postural retraining which, after the first year, were by far the most helpful. But all this time I was receiving a disability pension from the NFB. I was just plain lucky to be among the last filmmakers hired as staff, with full union benefits. My friends who started working at the NFB as freelancers a few months later than I—Terre, Gerry, Sidonie—would not have been covered. In another country, another time, with a less affluent or less supportive family, I could have been left at any of the stages through which I passed in my recuperation.

I shudder that Rosalie was sent home from brain surgery to teach herself to walk while I received so much professional rehabilitation therapy. She reminds me that the nightmare of being sick or disabled in most places in the world is to fall into irrevocable poverty.

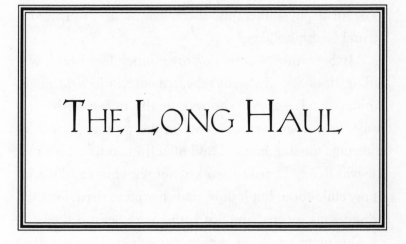

THE LONG HAUL

❧ Costa Rica ❧

After Michael had told Naomi that it was impossible for him to take me somewhere warm for the winter, an opportunity arose as if by magic. McGill University, where Michael was Professor of Family Medicine, received a request from the Costa Rican Ministry of Health for someone to help train teachers of family medicine. The job would run from January to March—perfect!

I was ready to go. *Mile Zero* was launched and flying on its own. Naomi was graduating with honors from her new *cégep*. Meena was going to work for a friend whose husband was home with Alzheimer's. Michel Danakas assured me that three months' vacation from my outpatient routine would only do me good. "Promise me you won't look for a physiotherapist there," he said. "You need a mental health holiday."

My big worry was leaving my mother. Her health was fading dramatically, with repeated infections and pneumonias. By December she was totally unresponsive, no smile, no recognition. She was on the waiting list for an end-stage nursing home. I told myself I had to accept that she was dying. I tried to awaken her with hugs and stories of my childhood, but it only made her more tired. I started bringing my journal and just sitting with her quietly.

One night I woke up writing her eulogy. The next day I went through all the steps of planning for her funeral, coolly typing out instructions until suddenly I realized what I was doing and cried.

In this uncertain state, Michael, Naomi, and I left Montreal. After two weeks vacation in Costa Rica, Naomi would fly home to wait tables at a yuppie dessert bar and apply to university, my typed list of funeral arrangements tucked in her suitcase.

Journal: January 3, 1989, Tamarindo
Last night I saw the sun set over the water, with a red afterglow reflecting on the sand, and Michael riding the waves, playing like a boy. How many times have I watched him do this? Today I swam in the ocean, going from hysteria at the smallest wave to what Michael called "inappropriate euphoria," floating over waves and trying to dive into them. I can almost kick, or at any rate I'm dragging my legs less and pulling better with my arms. I'm walking with canes on the packed sand, including bumpy

patches and inclines. I'm still choking, but less. I'm staying up
later at night. I hardly bite my tongue at all.

Journal: January 11, 1989
Last night Michael and Naomi went to spy on egg-laying Leath-
erback turtles, a long inaccessible walk to a secluded beach.
Michael felt bad to go without me, especially as I had a momentary cry at dinner because the restaurant had a giant step
at the front and everyone stared as he and Naomi hauled me
up by the armpits. After, Michael asked, "Are you scared?"

"Of what?" I answered.

But we both knew: scared of not getting better. I told him
I'm not scared—I can't afford to be. And if *he's* scared, I don't
want to know about it.

This morning I'm sitting on the beach, writing. Naomi and
Michael have gone walking again and I feel trapped in the
wheelchair, unable to negotiate a move away from the sun in
this soft sand. I'm pleased that they know how to meet their
own needs, including the need to get away from me. But I can't
help resenting their ability to forget me, to walk as far as the
beach beckons, to explore without constraints. The anguish is
profound when I let it surface. It's always there and releases at
the slightest invitation. Joy is equally there: it's not just a cover-
up to keep the pain down. That's the emotional roller coaster of
my days, my hours.

I've been left on the beach for what seems like well over an
hour now. I'm frying in the sun. I haven't stretched. I'm afraid to
stand because I fell once in the restaurant already this morning. I don't want to end up on the ground with sand blowing in

my face. There are people around who would surely help me, but I'm feeling timid, ashamed to always be asking for help. Besides I don't feel like being "handled" by strangers.

My sun hat has blown off and I can't reach it to keep it from blowing further. I signal for help to a man standing nearby. His wife, further down the beach, clearly sees me but can't get his attention so she gives up and ignores me. At least I have suntan lotion and my journal. At least I don't have to go to the toilet.

Journal: January 17, 1989, San José
This is my BIG FIRST DAY ALONE! Another marker in my climb to "normalcy" and I've been looking forward to it. Michael left at 6 a.m. to begin his first day of work. It's my first day of work too; starting the book I decided to write about my stroke and recovery. I was planning to use the solitude to recover some memories of my second stroke: the optimism of our anniversary, followed by the fast slide into total paralysis. I have no real memories of that time, only other people's stories. My plan is to interview everyone—family, friends, health-care providers—and integrate their memories into the book. I need to find my own as well; the lost months are like a weight in my chest, and now that I've set myself up to dig for whatever remains, I'm afraid to start. I don't want to relive that terror, not here alone. Maybe I need to start more slowly, one tentative toe at a time instead of diving right in.

On Saturday, we went to a party for the Costa Rican family practice residents Michael is training, at the country cottage of one of the doctors. I'd been looking forward to meeting people who didn't know me before. No comparisons, no "She used to be a filmmaker" or "You must miss tennis." Just what *is*, now.

Michael lugged my chair from the car and I managed the front steps on canes. I could see that some people were shocked. They didn't expect what they saw. They all knew Michael, of course, but they didn't know anything about me. They had no idea what was wrong with me or if I'd been like this all my life. A few of the young residents came up immediately and introduced themselves. There were several children who seemed afraid of my chair at first, but they melted when I rang the Mickey Mouse bell. The others kept their distance, sipping drinks, playing soccer, and dancing. One woman told Michael the next day that she thought he and I were like brother and sister. My paranoid translation was, "What's a handsome man like you doing with a crippled wife?" But maybe it was a compliment in terms of our similarity, our compatibility. Or maybe all Jews look alike.

After a while, Michael asked me to dance. It was my first time dancing in public. I imagine we were quite a sight, but I didn't care. It's the miracle of disinhibition, as Gérald Godin would say.

Exhilarated, I asked one of the residents to dance. He showed me a new step that took a lot of fine foot control, and I was laughing and clutching his shirt. Then one of Michael's teaching colleagues asked me to dance. I was totally wiped out, but it was great!

Michael was across the room by then, talking with a group of government officials and hospital administrators. He wheeled me over but once I was there, the administrators would only talk to Michael. They were up on a step and I was down in the wheelchair, but they didn't move any closer. They totally ignored me. They were even talking *about* me, in the third person, as if I wasn't there. At one point, I moved my chair right in front of them. I was obviously saying "I want to be part of this group and get to know you guys." But they continued their conversation, eyes averted. Even now, four days later I can hardly write about it. When I left they didn't say goodbye.

By the time Michael came to bed I was a quivering mess and I blurted out all that I was feeling. "Why should you be burdened with me?" I asked. "This isn't what you bargained for when we got married!" He replied that I was exactly the same person he had married and that it was the best decision of his life.

Journal: February 8, 1989, San José
Yesterday we discovered a woman who does both massage and acupuncture, so today I awoke revived and energetic. I took down the laundry from the clothesline, holding onto the wobbly rope with one hand, removing the clothes pin with the other, and valiantly attempting to catch each falling item before it hit the dirt. I've come to see the pleasure as well as the boredom in housework. I linger over tasks I used to do as fast as I could, while my mind was working on something "important." Nowadays, cleaning a papaya or cutting strawberries is an activity unto itself with its own aesthetic. I've had to learn to accept how long everything takes. Even now, when I fight it or forget it, my body rebels; I scramble my words, stumble and fall. I have to listen to what my body is telling me. It's not negotiable.

Journal: February 10, 1989, San José
Seth is coming tomorrow for two whole weeks. And the day

after Seth arrives Michael is going back to Montreal for three weeks. My excitement at seeing Seth is almost drowned out by my fear of spending a week all by myself in the new apartment we will be moving to.

I've been trying to see it as a challenge, another step on the road back to normalcy. But today I've been alone since Michael went to work at eight, and I've been watching the clock since noon. How will I last a whole week without human contact and specifically without him?

I'm having trouble with my total dependence on Michael. He is so tactful, fun, and uncomplaining. But on the rare moments when he indicates fatigue or—rarer still—irritability, I break up. And then he feels terrible. The other day I had to cross over some freshly-watered lawn to get to the apartment. I couldn't take my sneakers off or scrape them while standing, so I tracked mud through the room to get to a chair. Michael's uncensored horror made me feel like a naughty child.

He's been having back trouble again—we're not sure why. I wish I could help Michael. I wish I could tell him to go to bed and let me do the shopping, take the car for a tune-up, make dinner. I keep replaying our conversation about aging. Whenever Michael's back acts up like this, I know he's thinking about the future, worrying about not being in shape to help me.

I *have* to get better.

Journal: February 13, 1989, Cahuita
I lay in bed this morning, torturing myself with unanswerable questions. If Michael died or left me, how would I survive? Old age could be pretty horrible. Why do I get in a knot about these

what-if scenarios? I have recurring nightmares that a tumor is forming anew in the water-filled space we saw as a black hole in last October's MRI; or that there is a parallel malformation on the other side, which somehow no one noticed. I must not let myself dwell on these things. I don't know how I'll be doing next month, let alone in twenty years. Life is out of our control, no matter what illusions we carry.

Tape: February 14, 1989
Bonnie: This is CR tape No. 6. We're in Cahuita, a tropical rainforest in Costa Rica, and the date is February 14. Happy Valentine's Day!
Seth: It's the anniversary of the day you came home from the Institut.
Bonnie: Yes. I should be exhilarated. But instead I'm crying.
Seth: Do you want to turn off the tape?
Bonnie: No, let's just keep going. What was I crying about? Oh right—the Institut. I cry about everything these days. You probably noticed how irritable I was with Michael before he left.
Seth: Well . . . yes.
Bonnie: I guess it was hard to miss. I phoned him in Montreal last night to apologize for making his departure so awful. Michael wondered if I was nervous about seeing you. I could tell from the way my stomach clenched up that it was true. Because for a long time, whenever you came home for the weekend, you were always so excited about the progress I'd made since you last saw me, even if it was just the week before. And this time it had been six whole weeks! I wanted to show you lots of progress, but instead I realized how little has changed.

Seth: Six weeks is a short time.

Bonnie: What did you expect to find? Did you expect me to be further along?

Seth: No. I thought it would be pretty much the same.

Bonnie: When you picture me—when you just imagine me or think of Mom, do you picture me as I am now or as I was before the stroke?

Seth: I guess it varies. But usually when I imagine you, it's neither. When I imagine you, it's not doing stuff, it's sitting and talking. So there's nothing to say it was before or after.

Bonnie: You think of me as talking, not doing?

Seth: No, it's just that those quiet talking times have been important, ever since I was a little kid and I'd crawl into bed with you and Dad and tell you everything I was thinking about. And we still do it. Just before you left for Costa Rica, we were all lying around, and I was telling you how hard the tour year was, and how much better I felt this year.

Bonnie: And you were surprised when I said this year had been the best one of my life too.

Journal: February 19, 1989, San José
This morning was the first time in a year and a half that I've slept in an empty house and woken up alone. I've been dreading this moment for weeks, but now that it's arrived, I'm thrilled.

I made coffee and cereal with fresh bananas and strawberries, and then I wheeled outside into the amazing accessible garden, and sat under the bougainvillea tree, with the wind in the branches and the hollow thump of a basketball next door. All I missed was the *Sunday Times*.

Until now, I wasn't ready to remember the painful details of the stroke. But Costa Rica has given me the time and perhaps the distance I needed, and now every day new memories startle into consciousness. Lying on a stretcher in the JGH hallway, waiting for some test. Razelle crying. The smell of the supplement. Naomi arguing with the Hun. I write them down as they come. Write an hour, cry an hour: that's my routine.

The neighborhood is moving into evening. A flock of parrots squawks by and I have a perfect view of their symmetrical colors. The monkeys' happy hour is in shrieking progress. I hear doors opening, people calling to each other.

The sun is going down now and I'm thinking about dinner. I know from experience that I have to take care of my hunger before it makes me crazy, but I don't want to miss the sunset. So, a conflict between two loves—how to resolve it? I think I can have both if I walk to the kitchen and fix myself something I can carry back out to the garden, but I don't have any pockets, so how will I carry it? I could put peanut butter on bread and carry it in my mouth but I might choke. I could wrap it around one cane handle so I can kind of hold it and walk at the same time. But which way should I wrap it—so the peanut butter squishes on the cane or my hand? Or I can carry it in my knapsack. That's what I'll do. Perfect solution. Here I go.

OK, here's the denouement we've all been waiting for. I peeled a hard boiled egg, sliced a tomato, buttered some bread, made up a sandwich, all leaning on the counter. Made a big mess. Then wrapped it up in a napkin, tucked it into a plastic bag, put it into my knapsack and trundled out to catch the last five minutes of light. And a hard-boiled egg sandwich never tasted better.

Journal: February 21, 1989, San José
I'm amazed at how well I'm doing, doing nothing. The days simply unfold. Even days that are empty of plans are full of
surprises. I think I'm learning how to live.

Today I got smart and dragged my exercise mat into the
garden. I was able to hear the birds and the basketball and
smell the orange blossoms. I felt completely relaxed, not rushing through my exercises but exploring them. I'm beginning to
combine what I remember of yoga with Emilie's unstructured
movement, Judith's Feldenkrais, and Michel's physio, in a routine that's no longer Emilie's or Judith's or Michel's, but mine,
improvised to suit my body from the inside out.

Yesterday I was looking through the gate at the garden: the
gardenia, the wild orchids, the purple azalea. Front and center
was my black wheelchair; this unnatural machine, hard and
shiny, plastic and steel, spoiling the landscape. I hate it. I realized I've been feeling like I too spoil the landscape, making
people uncomfortable just by being there. But today on the
mat I reclaimed my right to be a part of nature. Too bad if
people can see me through the gate. It's good for them to see
me and see how hard I work. It's not ugly, it's life.

Journal: March 1, 1989, San José
Michael's return Thursday evening was disappointing. He immediately got busy trying to fix the computer instead of making
love. I felt ugly and unsexy, even though he claimed that the
problem was his and not mine.

This evening when Michael and I danced, I was weepy. Because he had been outside playing basketball—*my* girlhood

sport—while I was curled up in bed. And because what I do is hardly dancing, and dancing was one of the fun things we did together, starting the day we met, twenty-two years ago. I want to kick up my heels and THEY WON'T GO, dammit!

Journal: March 6, 1989, San José
Michael got sick yesterday. He woke in the middle of the night and went to the bathroom. The next thing I knew he crawled back across the floor and collapsed. I didn't know what to do. I couldn't even help him get up onto the bed. I pulled the covers over him and he whimpered himself to sleep. He was better in a few hours. We figured it was some kind of food poisoning; still, it was a flash of his mortality.

Ever since that incident, we've been close and loving. I guess it startled us into remembering what's important.

Journal: March 10, 1989, San José
This morning Michael and I lay in bed and talked for hours. In the end, he decided he has to resign as Chief of Family Medicine and Director of the Herzl Family Practice Center. He's worn out from over fourteen years of fighting the same political battles at the JGH where expensive specialty medicine is valued more than the kind of integrated care which Michael practices and teaches. He will still do childbirth research and look after patients—the part of his work which he enjoys the most. But not being Director will give him the time and space to see what he wants to do next. We talked about the possibility of moving to a more disability-friendly city with better weather and accessible transit. Michael, who is so committed to his work, has

consistently put it second to my recovery. He continues to surprise me—I think he surprises himself.

While Michael was settling into this tough decision about his own work, I played filmmaker for the first time since we've been in Costa Rica, showing *Speaking Our Peace* at the Friends' Peace Center. The audience was appreciative and full of questions, and my voice stayed strong, with only a few choking spells.

It was strange seeing myself in the film. Michael said he had forgotten my old voice. Watching the film, I remembered being at the women's peace camp at Greenham Common, surrounded by police with guns and dogs; then at the Eldorado nuclear facility, under police surveillance for asking questions about nuclear contamination. And in the Soviet Union, the film authorities, who were linked to the KGB, were incensed about an interview I'd taped, in Hebrew, with a Jewish refusenik. They called me in, alone, on the eve of our departure, and physically erased the tape. I was the only one, in this room of Soviet film apparatchiks, who understood the disappearing words. It was the worst moment of my filmmaking life, to hear a voice silenced as I stood by, powerless.

People have been reassuring me that I'll be able to make films again. No one is more surprised than I to find out that I can live quite well without that role. At the same time I do remember how satisfying it is. So, while I cavalierly say "I don't need to make films any more," last night I experienced it as a loss.

Journal: March 23, 1989, Samara
In a little more than a week we'll be in Montreal. I've made dra-

matic progress in the last few weeks, after several months of
invisible build up. I feel it as sure-footedness, more trust that
my legs will hold me, that the ground won't shift as I step. I can
walk without total concentration, with fewer of those missteps
that make every move tentative. I'm standing straighter and,
when I remind myself, I can look ahead as I walk instead of at
my feet! It all comes together only when I'm perfectly rested
and relaxed, but it's enough to see that it can and *will* come together in time. Michel Danakas was right. I've become
"de-institutionalized."

Journal: March 25, 1989, Samara
We called Montreal this morning. Mom is in the hospital again
with pneumonia. Naomi feels they caught it early enough and
it's under control for the moment, but she is worried. I couldn't
have come to Costa Rica if Naomi were not watching over
Mom. I wonder if she knows what an enormous, unspeakable
gift she has given me.

   My feelings unfold slowly with the news. Horror that my
mother's body is not letting her die when she has been waiting
so long. Guilt that I have prolonged the wait for my own convenience, for if I were there I think we would simply withhold the
treatment that keeps forcing her back. It's a bitter irony that I've
been writing about how much it means to have a loved one beside you touching you, and I haven't been there for my own
mother. Now I can only pray that she does hold on long enough
so that I can say what she may need to hear. I don't know exactly what words to use, but I'm sure they'll come if I'm
fortunate enough to be with her again. Maybe she needs to

hear that she loved us and took good care of us, as we love her and are taking care of her now. Maybe she needs to know it's OK to let go and die.

Journal: April 2, 1989, Montreal
Mom looked shrunken and pale, but didn't seem uncomfortable. The room reeked of the nutritional supplement. When I tried to unclench her fist to hold her hand, she reacted with what seemed like crying. Michael said, "That hurts her now," but I interpreted her reaction as anger at me for having gone away. After that, she was unresponsive, except for a feeble smile when Michael joked with her. I begged for some sign that she knew who I was. I heard myself "explain" my long absence, how much good it had done me, etc. But to empty eyes. I finally pressed her—"Are you angry with me because I left you?"—realizing how much, how selfishly and absurdly, I wanted to be forgiven by my mother, as she has always forgiven me.

Journal: April 10, 1989
On Sunday the nurse called to say my mother appeared to be going downhill fast, and we all rushed to the hospital. She was breathing heavily, and her hands were blue. Her eyes were unfocused, as they'd been most of the week. She still seemed peaceful. We held her hands and stroked her head. When I told her that Naomi was there, she made her only volitional move—she turned her head to look, focused clearly, and reached out her hand for Naomi's. I was pleased that her last gesture before she died was towards her granddaughter who had stood vigil in my place.

❀ Spring, 1989 ❀

Spring, one-and-a-half years PS (post-stroke). How do I write about this time? The landmarks are fuzzy, the time-frame blurs as days melt into weeks and months and nothing much changes. Progress is measured by being able to stand upright for one minute longer in a month's time, or to walk on canes another twenty feet, or to ride on the stationary bike for so many more seconds at such-and-such resistance. But the urgency to recover is no less, the desperate need to be how and who I was before a weakened knot of blood vessels bisected my life. I want clear answers, steady progress towards a concrete goal, but the will-she/won't-she slow dance of rehabilitation gives me only uncertainty.

Journal: April 27, 1989

A few days ago, one of my Studio D friends called to ask if I was going to the Canadian Women's Film Festival in Israel next month. I was embarrassed to admit that no one had told me about it, despite the fact that they're screening both Not a Love Story and Speaking Our Peace. I was especially frustrated because Michael and I are going to Israel a few weeks later—he has a conference and a month-long visiting professorship in Beer Sheva. If I had known, we might have been able to leave in time for the film festival.

Then, yesterday, as I was sitting in the front hall, waiting for the Transport Adapté to take me for my first session back at the Institut, the festival organizer called. One of the invited film-makers had to cancel—would I like to attend? My immediate response was anger—why hadn't she invited me in the first place? Now Michael has commitments he can't rearrange in order to go two weeks earlier. She didn't seem to understand that I can't travel alone.

She told me they needed an answer right away, in order to find someone else if necessary. So, with the Transport Adapté beeping its horn in my driveway, I turned down an opportunity that likely won't recur—a coming together of three of my previous passions: women, film, and Israel.

At the Institut, the halls were lined with people slumped in wheelchairs. The carpets stank of stale smoke. There was no one I wanted to see. Michel Danakas sprained his back lifting a quadriplegic patient twice his size, and is away on a one-year disability leave. Judith is on holiday. With that news, I decided not to return to the outpatient program. Why go through all the Institut hassle in order to work with strangers? I will seek out my own therapists.

I had another frustrating forty minute wait for the Transport Adapté in the smoky lobby. Finally, I made my way up the stairs to the house, miserable. Naomi was coming out on her way to work. She hugged me and I poured out my woes: I don't want to be handicapped—it's lousy and it's lasting forever. I hate the Institut and the Transport Adapté. And I can't go to the film festival because I can't travel alone! When Naomi heard the whole story she offered to quit her job a month early and go with me.

I called the festival organizer immediately, only to learn she'd offered the trip to someone else who is thinking about it overnight! I should have been more assertive in the first call. Why didn't I ask for some time to consider? When Michael came home, he brushed aside my self-blame and suggested Naomi and I go anyway, despite the expense. "Why do you need to be officially sponsored?" he asked. I had no answer, but in my heart I still wish I had that validation.

At my pre-trip check-up, Joe Carlton congratulated my decision to go to the festival, saying, "It's time to resume your life, and come to terms with where you are now."

I walked out of his office swallowing my tears. Was he, my would-be tennis partner, telling me it was time to give up and accept my greatly-reduced physical status?

❦ Israel ❦

Naomi: As soon as we got to the baggage claim area in Ben Gurion airport, my mother announced, "Everyone looks like my cousin."

It's true, they did. Black kinky hair, olive skin, lots of emotions. Even the hippyish flowing clothing is the kind my mother loves. Like a family reunion only you don't know anyone.

That was the problem with Israel. Our hopes were too high and the trip was doomed from the start. This was a voyage to the homeland but my mother had been rejected before we even arrived. Grudgingly invited, then disinvited, then made to pay her own way. But once we got to Israel, Mom was a media star. Her picture was in the major Hebrew newspaper and she was on the Israeli equivalent of *60 Minutes. Not a Love Story* was the sensation of the festival, more screenings had to be scheduled, more press conferences, more discussion groups.

The festival organizers seemed to resent it. They planned parties and "forgot" to invite us. They didn't sit with us in the theaters. We didn't even eat together. Within a day of our arrival, it became pretty clear that Mom and I were on our own in Israel; no one was going to help us out. It seemed as if her disability was a big inconvenience: she wasn't just showing them up, she was slowing them down. The festival was a turning point in my mother's recovery. It was her first big trip without Dad since her stroke, her re-entry into the world of film. She should have been made to feel like a hero because it was a truly momentous and joyful occasion. Instead she was made to feel like a drag.

Journal: May 22, 1989

I can no longer move in what used to be my world. The organizers had promised to "accommodate" me, but instead I'm expected to fit in and keep up. It's as if I've been used for my films and my name, but made invisible as a person. I feel the festival organizers are ashamed of me because I no longer project the feminist ideals of strength, competence, and independence. An Amazon I'm not—I can't even fake it.

Naomi: *Not a Love Story* not only upstaged the other women's films, it upstaged my mother's other, more recent films like *Speaking Our Peace* and *Mile Zero*. The Israelis were having the porn debate with all the emotion and fervor that North Americans had ten years before. Women wept. Men screamed. The media went nuts.

The strangest thing was hearing my mother's narration in the first five minutes of the film. The woman next to me leaned over and asked, "Is that your mother talking?" I said "No, I think she got somebody else to read it." It wasn't

until the end of the film that I realized it *was* her voice—
her old voice.

Journal: May 24, 1989
Watching Not a Love Story after so many years, I see that it's really about voice—or lack of it. The dialogue about pornography and erotica has evolved since 1981 and become more complex, but Not a Love Story was part of breaking women's silence, opening our eyes and our mouths. Seeing it now in Israel, I realize the coherence of my life's work. It wasn't a series of unrelated films, but variations on a related theme: speech vs. silence, solidarity vs. isolation, peace vs. violence.

Naomi: It was the first year of the *intifadah* (Palestinian uprising) and much as the tourism department tried to play it down, Israel was a country at war. The news was filled with reports of random bombings and shootings, and, as always, the streets were filled with eighteen-year-old boys carrying Uzis.

Our hotel was on a hill in the outskirts of Jerusalem. We couldn't go anywhere without scaling a sixty-degree slope which my mother couldn't begin to wheel by herself in her manual chair. Besides, the black metal wheel rims were too hot from the summer heatwave to even touch.

People responded to us in two ways: with total indifference, as from taxi drivers who popped their trunks, refusing to get out of their cars to help me load and unload the wheelchair; or with totally overbearing and intrusive "help." If we were having trouble getting up a curb or out of a cab, passersby would physically push me aside and manhandle my mother, often lifting the wheelchair with her in it without asking her permission. Yes, everyone looks like your cousin, but they also act like they own you—as only families can.

The trip to Israel was supposed to be a show of independence for my mother and of adult responsibility for me, and we both were failing. Without my Dad's legitimizing presence, it became clear that the "you can do anything" feeling that my mother had up until our trip was slipping away. I just couldn't give it to her. It seemed that everything about the country—the landscape, the climate, the people, the ground itself—was conspiring to make disability more difficult.

Journal: May 27, 1989

I had a moment of crying in the bank today. Naomi was upstairs getting some money changed, and I was in line to cash a traveler's check. I think it was the waiting. No, it was the aloneness in the wheelchair, and the realization of how much I hate it. I don't want to become wheelchair-independent—to go out among the crowds and curbs with no one I can count on but myself. It's a hard admission: I want to be taken care of.

Later I swam and exercised in the water—better, harder, and longer than ever before. Sometimes despair leads to depression. Sometimes it can be motivating. People call this "courage," but it's not that. It's just the desire to heal, to get on with living as I wish to live, to see our children's lives unfold. Naomi says I'll find new energy once I settle into wherever I do land physically. She offers no promises of total recovery, just the observation that it's been a very long time, that I'm sick of being sick, and that I'm still recovering. I don't fully understand what she means but I feed off her optimism. I keep wondering if true acceptance means to stop challenging myself to do things as I used to, which was exhausting even when I was "normal," and avoid the frustrating comparisons with Before. Maybe "independence" is a misleading concept. Each of us is dependent on others. Perhaps independence is not the ultimate goal, but interdependence: the possibility of doing with and for each other, the ability to ask for the help that we each need.

❈ Montreal ❈

Journal: July 10, 1989

I've been feeling down ever since we got home. I seem to have lost that incredible sense of aliveness, of living-on-the-edge.

We were so high that first post-stroke year. The lows were correspondingly low, but it was an intense experience filled with love and discovery. But now, near the end of the second year, reality has sunk in. I'm constantly confronted by all the things I can no longer do. My progress is barely measurable. Anyone watching me walk would see struggle and pain. I lean heavily on the canes. My knees are rigidly locked, making my back hyper-extended. My right hip sinks back and my shoulders corkscrew in opposite directions. My gait is broad, with the right foot dragging and slapping down. My eyes stare at my feet. On the rare occasions when I look up and catch a glimpse of myself in a mirror or window, I look like a robot.

I can no longer regard this as a passing phase. Normal life has resumed for Michael and my other loved ones, but I'm still not normal. I swore I would never again take life for granted, but now I have whole days where I can't wait for night to come so I can collapse on my bed.

Summer dragged by. In September, Naomi and Seth left for the University of Toronto. I spent the last weeks before they went in what was to become a familiar pattern: telling myself to enjoy the time we had, and then spoiling that time by clinging. The day they left, I was determined to be brave and not make them feel bad. Seth woke early and made them both sandwiches. Later I tortured myself, thinking: that's what a Real Mom would have been doing instead of tossing through a sleepless night. The car was stuffed, mostly with Naomi's things. She'd been rummaging for weeks in our basement for objects to beautify her dorm room. I gave her a crystal to hang in her window, with a quote from the poem she had written two years before: "I give to you now / what you have given to me . . . "

Seth and I had said goodbye many times over the past three years. But this was Naomi's first year away from home, and my first year with both our children gone. Our goodbye was an intense mix of exuberance and sadness. Naomi was beaming as she said, "I'm sorry." Sorry she's leaving? Sorry she's growing up? Sorry for past sins? "I'm not sorry," I told her, which was a lie. I was drowning in regrets and self-pity, remembering all the times I was unavailable to Naomi. When she was little she would sometimes call my office after school, bored and lonely, and ask me what she could do. I was often too busy to talk for long. When I had to go away for a film shoot, she would say "Don't go Mummy!"

Now it was I who needed her, and she who was busy with her life. I didn't know how to behave. I desperately wanted to ask her if I'd been a good mother to her, but I restrained myself. I wanted to be generous about letting go, but my heart had not stopped grieving. My losses were interconnected: I mourned my mother, my daughter, my future, my self.

Journal: September 27, 1989
I feel like Michael and I are at a stage in life where little will be new. We've got the mid-life, empty-nest blahs. I notice how much more we laughed with the kids around, how much intellectual stimulation their daily presence gave our lives. I've been taping interviews with friends, but I wonder if it's just an empty exercise for a book I'll never write. I find myself tuning out ideas that once absorbed me. I have subscriptions to all the same magazines, but now I put them aside, unopened. It scares me. Feminism gave me a way to understand my place in the world, but I don't seem to belong there any more. I don't know where I belong.

As Autumn settled in, my depression intensified. I was still too weak—and too nervous—to go out alone, and even in good weather organizing someone to go with me often seemed more trouble than it was worth. My friends were busy with their own lives and work. I remember one trip to my local grocery store pushed by Eileen, a young woman who'd been transcribing my journals. It was my first time there since the stroke, and I was thrilled with the smell of fresh bread, the familiar trout swimming in their murky tank, the chickens barbecuing. I felt good to be buying lunch and dinner for Michael—Meena was home with a cold and besides I wanted to wean my dependence on her. I smiled to the familiar clerks and got nothing but cold stares. The cashier, a woman I'd seen for years, didn't recognize me, so she called the manager to verify my check. Fair enough, I thought. The manager asked for a driver's license. As I was fumbling for my old one (cancelled since my stroke), feeling bad for the people waiting behind, I explained to him that I'd been a customer for over ten years.

"I have to ask for this—it's a formality," he responded, looking at Eileen. I thought he must be cross-eyed—always giving the benefit of the doubt. Why else would he address Eileen when I was there talking to him, obviously competent. So I answered that I understood, and he again spoke to Eileen, unmistakably, referring to me in the third person: "She won't have to show it next time, once we know her. It's the rules." There was no next time.

Journal: October 15, 1989

In my ongoing push to resume "real life," I've been trying to add more social exercise to my rehab routine—with mixed success. I had a delicious swim at our local YMCA pool yesterday; then I fell in the shower room. It was maddening because I had asked them to get non-slip matting around the pool and in the shower. According to the director, they used to have some, but it started to stink from chlorine and they threw it out. Sure enough one of my canes slipped on the wet floor, and I did a slow-motion fall. Luckily I wasn't hurt or bruised, but every fall brings the threat of breaking a bone, creating even greater limitation. By the time I was dressed and leaving, the executive director had sent word that she will be sure mats are purchased next week. I'm optimistic they will be, if only for fear of liability, though it is hard not to hear echoes of the membership director who told Michael last month, "This is not a priority."

Last week I signed up for a course in t'ai chi for seniors. I've taken t'ai chi before, in my "old life," and liked it. I figured a seniors' class would be slow enough for me, and it might make me feel good to be taking an "almost normal" class instead of always having to go to special handicapped programs or not go at all. It might even make me feel graceful.

But when the time came, I couldn't do it. What was I thinking of? My self-image hasn't adjusted to this massive change at all. Did I imagine I could stand and sink down at my knees and shift my weight as I gracefully turned my body? I can't balance on two feet, let alone one. I spent the class listlessly doing the arm motions in my chair.

With no formal rehabilitation program, I was desperately seeking alternatives to keep up my motivation and hope. We researched nutritional supplements and added an array of vitamins and minerals, ginseng, and foul-tasting Chinese herbs to my daily regime. I never knew there were so many healers around, so many varieties of touch, massage, movement and dance. I tried everything, looking for the right match of teacher and method. After many trials and false starts I met Diane Genereux, a former physio who

now taught Feldenkrais, the method to which Judith
Blumberger introduced me when I was still at the Institut.
Twice a week Diane came to my house. One session was
for hands-on floor work, in which her hands gently guided
me to an awareness of how I used my body, especially where
I held tension. The other session was more active, with a
series of subtle movements that I visualized before perform-
ing. I learned to move with the least amount of effort. The
aim of this work was not to regain lost functions but to
maximize what I had through focus and awareness.

When I pushed her to tell me, Diane agreed with Michel
Danakas that my walking still wasn't functional, but suggested I use one cane as a bridge to walking free. That would
mean I could carry things in my other hand—a huge step
forward—my first really tangible step in months. I couldn't
wait to show Michael! In a burst of enthusiasm, I hid my
second cane in the back of the hall closet and wore myself
out (and smashed several dishes) trying to make dinner all
by myself. The freedom of one cane was counterbalanced
by exhaustion and muscle pain—a poor trade-off. The other
cane came back out of the closet—just for longer walks, I
told myself, just for awhile. But almost without noticing, I
slipped back into using two canes for everything.

~

As Fall slid into Winter, I was housebound for days at a
time. Michael and I walked around the block during a brief
break in the weather. It took the better part of an hour,
with Michael cheering me on, but I was steady on my canes,

never had to stop, and recovered after a twenty-minute lie-down. I phoned Naomi to brag about my progress.

"You can walk!" she crowed.

"It's not real walking," I corrected her immediately, my moment of triumph dashed.

I continued to attempt "real" walking, without canes. It came in unpredictable, unrepeatable spurts, and when it came there was no stopping me.

Journal: November 5, 1989

Last night I got the urge, and I walked around our house without canes. I shifted my full weight with each step, and felt the floor with my feet. Michael and I sang to give me a good rhythm. When I felt as if I was falling, instead of grabbing at the wall, I corrected myself without panicking. I was stiff-kneed, with a wide gait, but I felt confident, surefooted and not dizzy. I screamed with joy, and so did Michael. "This means a full recovery!" he said. "It may take a few more years but nothing will stop you."

It's so mystical and absurd, this short circuit between my brain and my muscles. But moments like this give me a sense of what's possible, and I feel like dancing all the time.

There are no journal entries for the next day, no record of the inevitable letdown, Michael's steady encouragement hiding his disappointment, my waning effort, exhaustion, despair. Again and again I celebrated my "big breakthrough" only to see it slip from my grasp the next day. Each time, Michael celebrated with me, as convinced as I that this was it.

In late November, I went for my driver's test. The examination took place at the Lethbridge Rehabilitation Center in nearby Montreal West. It was the first time I had driven since my stroke. Once I had sat in our parked car, trying to shift from the gas to the brake, but my foot kept getting caught under the pedals. It didn't seem like I'd be safe going out on the road to practice, even with Michael (famed impatient driving instructor) beside me. But the Lethbridge Center had cars with hand controls for disabled drivers, and brakes for the instructors. Michael had encouraged me to try for my license in one of those. Once I learned to drive (and conquered my fear of going out alone and developed the strength to unload my wheelchair from the car and wheel myself from where I parked to where I wanted to go, or better yet learned to walk longer distances with or without canes), then I could start being truly independent.

So with no practice, in a heavy snowfall, I drove along Sherbrooke Street and didn't kill anyone. I drove with regular foot controls until fatigue set in, then with hand controls until total panic set in and I begged the instructor to take me home. But I got a license! It was restricted to driving with an official handicapped driving instructor until I was reevaluated. But it was a start.

As I was leaving the Rehab Center I saw someone driving up on a motorized three-wheeled vehicle. I had never seen an electric scooter before. They didn't seem to exist on the streets of Montreal. The young man astride the scooter had a jaunty look, in control of his destiny and destination. When I got home, I called the Institut and inquired. Everyone was horrified at the idea. If I had a scooter, I would no longer work at learning to walk, and besides, it would be an admission of failure. No one wanted to talk further about it.

Journal: November 26, 1989
This weekend we moved all our Vermont furnishings to an accessible cottage at Black Lake in the lower Laurentians. The morning brought ice on the lake and the chattering of red squirrels and anxious jays at the birdfeeder. I rolled out of bed excited for the first time in weeks. Or is it months? I managed to walk on one cane from the kitchen to the living room, carrying a big bunch of grapes in an inelegant but unbreakable green plastic bowl. I arrived with glee to "serve" Michael, after all his unpacking and setting up the house. A small triumph tinged with the ironic awareness of how small it was indeed, to limp across a floor with an ugly bowl. My pretensions to grace and elegance are so thwarted. I can't believe I ever felt like a dancer.

Journal: December 3, 1989
Yesterday I awoke with the first light showing Black Lake white and frozen. I wanted to run out and play in the snow, but instead I did my exercises by the window. All the various paths—physio, Feldenkrais, Emilie's continuum—are leading to the same place. I concentrate on feeling the floor under my feet, trusting my legs to bear my weight. I hear myself saying many times a day, "It's coming. It will come."

As I finished my workout, Michael walked in, wearing his corduroys and gaiters, ready for the first cross-country ski of the year. It was as if the image bypassed my brain and went straight to my heart. I didn't want to mar Michael's joy so I went to the bedroom with my tears. I watched him through the window, skiing down to the lake with Lucy ecstatically nipping at his heels.

I feel a pressure to hide my emotions—something inside telling me, "Control yourself for the sake of those who love you, and whom you need to keep loving you!" But whether I'm explicit about my feelings or not, those who love me end up having their happiness tinged with my loss.

Today was bright, beautiful, and freezing cold, and I woke up determined to go out and enjoy it. Michael pulled me down the hill in a plastic sled, with the snow flying in my face. Then, on the flat lake, I was able to walk on the snowshoes we gave Annie years ago. I used ski poles instead of canes. Again tears, but this time for joy.

We were in the country when Anne Usher called. "Are you watching TV? Do you know what's going on?"

It was impossible to believe. There was some man inside Montreal's Ecole Polytechnique shooting engineering students—all women. He said they were feminists taking jobs from men and he shot them. I thought that kind of thing only happened in the United States. This was Canada, Montreal, our home. I passed the Polytechnique on the way to the Institut when I was an outpatient. Where was Naomi? Was she safe in Toronto? Was she scared?

I felt so isolated. I no longer had a regular women's group, as I'd had with Studio D, with whom to strategize and scream. I wanted to go to the women's candlelight vigil but it was late on a freezing December night and no one knew whether it would be accessible. For the first time, I felt disconnected from the community of women. I had no one with whom to mourn.

❋ Winter ❋

Journal: February 10, 1990

We're en route to Israel where Michael will be instructing teachers of family medicine as he did in Costa Rica. I began this trip feeling happy and calm, even healthy. The preparation was relaxed and the kids in good shape, clearly ready to resolve their own problems. I'm looking forward to some time alone with Michael, and perhaps finding the energy to buckle down to work on my book.

El Al sat us far from the bathroom in spite of our requests—something about security not letting them assign seats in advance. It was 11:30 p.m., when I'm usually asleep, and I had to walk to the next cabin to get to the toilet. The aisles were too narrow for canes. I did fine in the forward direction, using the seat backs to hold and propel me forward, with Michael stabilizing me from behind. I was almost swinging along. But on the way back I had to face all those people, who couldn't help staring at me as I grabbed over their heads for their seat backs. I worked hard to avoid their eyes, to look stoic and dignified. When I finally reached my seat, I tried to hide my tears from Michael but he saw them and urged me to tell him what was happening. Usually he knows without words, so if he doesn't, it's only fair that I try to explain; we are living this together. I heard myself saying all sorts of reasonable things, like the trip is forcing me to face how disabled I still am. But then I blurted out what must be the deeper truth: all those people were staring at me, pitying me, and I hate it. I hate them for being normal while I'm not.

Michael listened, heard me out, then said, "They were staring at *me*. They're jealous because you're so beautiful." It sounds ridiculous now, but it was so incredibly sweet, and I think he believes it, though of course I do not.

Journal: February 13, 1990
I'm looking at the Sinai mountains, shrouded with history, and thinking how absurdly wonderful it is that we're here for Michael to *dive*—a week of pure pleasure before Beer Sheva and work. Michael is ecstatic with the Red Sea, and I'm pleased to share it. This morning was my best snorkel ever. Michael towed me, like he used to tow Naomi before she was a big swimmer, and I lasted over half an hour. I wore a pair of clear plastic beach shoes that kept me from fearing the fire coral and sea urchins as I still don't have an accurate sense of where my body is, especially my limp legs.

I'm walking quite well in the water and I can balance with the tide. I'm generally more stable on my feet. I walk further distances with my canes over incredible obstacles—flagstone paths, stony beaches, uneven sand—right into the water.

But yesterday's boat trip was exhausting. We were both muscle-sore afterwards, me from the boat crashing against the waves in a headwind. I had my usual pre-menstrual bout of jealousy—this time over a diver-doctor from Outremont. I was sure Michael would find her attractive. She was an emergentologist, shared his passion for scuba diving, did avalanche rescue, and was just back from horseback-riding Arabian stallions in Egypt! But Michael was considerably less interested than I was. I hate this in myself.

Journal: February 22, 1990
In the pattern of fear leading to determination, I worked very hard in the pool. I walked a narrow line of tiles, concentrating on placing the heel of my right foot before the ball. Then I did barre exercises at the deep end, trying to move my legs with slow control. Suddenly I glimpsed myself from outside: a crazy woman doggedly trying to force her spastic foot to respond to her will.

Until now, I have believed that I will get better with hard work and the passage of time. In the pool I suddenly wondered if I am stubbornly and stupidly fighting a losing battle, refusing to accept a reality which must seem obvious to everyone but me. I've been accused before of idealistically thinking I could change the world. But I don't want to accept being handicapped. What's the difference between acceptance and giving up?

Journal: March 12, 1990
I received a call from a member of the local chapter of the Israeli Women's Network. She asked me if, as a visiting feminist, I would speak at their next meeting on the "women's issue" of my choice.

My immediate response was no, I am no longer engaged with women's issues. I have nothing of interest to say to feminists. I don't even think of myself as a feminist any more. I've been absorbed, even obsessed, with my own body for the last two and a half years.

"That's exactly what we want to know about, but we were too shy to ask," she replied.

It was a small group gathered in someone's living room. I had forgotten how wonderful it is to talk intimately with a group of women! Though I barely knew them, I somehow felt safe. I read random bits from my journals—the first time I had shared them. My stories prompted theirs, and we heard each other's fears about our bodies, health, and aging. Our aloneness or our dependence. Our ability to survive. We realized we rarely talk about illness and suffering, disability and dying, though we will all confront these human realities. As we talked, I remembered how I used to insist that every issue is a women's issue. Maybe I'm still a feminist after all.

By the end of the evening I felt connected as I haven't for a long time. But I was also aware that no one else at the meeting was disabled. For all our intimacy, I was still in some way Other. I was still alone.

❧ Interlude: New Reproductive and Genetic Technologies ❧

Journal: November 10, 1994
I roll into the opening session of the roundtable on New Reproductive and Genetic Technologies, co-sponsored by the DisAbled Women's Network of Canada and the National Action

Committee on the Status of Women (NRGTS, DAWN Canada, and NAC in acronym-speak). It's a historic coming together to explore the complex and emotional questions of genetic screening and eugenic abortion as they affect women's equality and freedom of choice, particularly women with disabilities.

On the stage are four women seated at a table: DAWN Canada's Joan Meister, who spearheaded this dialogue of mainstream feminists and women with disabilities; U.S. women's health and disability rights activist Marsha Saxton; Sunera Thobani, the chair of NAC, who will speak on the "contradictions of choice;" and a woman I have never seen before on a high bar chair at the end of the table, her bare feet crossed on the table. Her body is armless; a black silk shirt is stitched at the armholes, and she wears a flashy vest. My eyes are fixed on her animated form as she takes notes with one foot, stopping to lift a glass of water to her mouth. After each speaker, her feet clap.

Theresia Dagener is a lawyer and radical activist in Germany, well-versed in the history and ideology of eugenics. Theresia's disability is the result of Thalidomide, the wonder drug given to pregnant women in the late fifties and early sixties to prevent nausea, a walking warning of the fallibility of medical science.

Her position is clear: Abortion, Yes; New Reproductive and Genetic Technologies, No. She is not in favor of *laws* against the selective abortion of disabled fetuses, but neither does she consider such abortions to be acts of feminist self-determination.

"Most people, feminists included," she says, "just cannot imagine disability as a neutral condition, which is not necessarily linked with suffering or with happiness." Choosing to abort a disabled fetus is based on prejudice, the same as choosing to abort because the fetus is female. The problem is the lack of social support for people with disabilities and their families. The solution is to change society, not to eliminate people with disabilities. Disability is a part of human life; whether from illness, accidents, aging, environmental causes, or genetic differences.

What a smart move that the organizers of this roundtable did not invite the press. It seemed to me a wasted opportunity at first, but there's no way that we would have been so honest with each other. Marsha said that women have been forced to "dehumanize the fetus" to protect our right to choose abortion. The women at the roundtable were pro-choice, but their views are too complex for sound bites and polarized slogans to convey.

～

I can't sleep after the conference opening. My head is spinning with all I've learned. Multinational pharmaceutical companies, manufacturers of related equipment, and university medical research establishments all have huge financial investments in genetic technology. Most of us have been convinced that this technology will eliminate suffering and reduce the burden on families and society. "Science" will soon be able to create life without woman or man, and to shape that life to preconceived specifications of perfection. Eliminating everything undesirable, abnormal, *interesting*.

In the state between sleep and wakefulness, I find myself obsessing on Theresia—straining to remember exactly how she looked: What color were her eyes? Did she have empty sleeves or had she cut them off? Did she take notes and adjust the mike with the same foot?

What an effect she had on me. Is this what we mean by the "Power of Difference?"

I have a vision of Theresia, a torso on a rearing white horse, leading the troops like Joan of Arc. To where, against whom? She is joined in my vision by Marsha, who was born with spina bifida, a condition for which there are now prenatal tests; many pregnant women automatically abort. Other DAWN *women are in this army (our people), looking like all forms of fetus, with missing or undeveloped limbs, facial reconstruction for "birth defects." And I am there too, with my "congenital malformation" that cost the medical system so much to fix. "We are the living fetuses," I think.*

When I awake, my "censor" finds my dream melodramatic and grandiose. But I want to trust this vision of leadership by women who know in our own bodies the shortsightedness of technology, the arrogance of eugenic ideals of perfection, the hurtfulness of discrimination, the strength of survival. People with disabilities have unique perspectives on the meaning of human life.

COMING OUT

Journal: June 19, 1990

Nelson Mandela spoke in Montreal today. After my apolitical doldrums of last winter, I surprised myself with my eagerness to go hear him. It's his first time in Canada since his long imprisonment and I wanted to mark this event with my community. Anne Usher said she'd go with me, but was concerned about wheelchair access. So I began a day of inquiry. I ended up talking to someone at City Hall who was cordial, but obviously had never considered the question. They would research it and call back.

Hours later came a call from a regretful City Hall staffer: "I am very sorry but we are not able to make special arrangements for wheelchairs. Everyone will be standing, with all the media in the front. There will be no one to help you. All the streets will be closed. You have to take public transit, no cars or taxis. ("But *the Metro is totally inaccessible,*" I say to myself.)

"Mandela is next to the Pope's visit in terms of security,"
the staffer continues. (*"So God forbid someone with crutches wants to
see the Pope,"* I smart-ass silently.)

"We are sorry to say it, but perhaps the best thing would be
for you to watch on TV. Otherwise, come with at least two
friends, if they are healthy, (*could I have heard right?*) and arrive by
4:15 p.m. The streets are cobble-stoned, so it will be difficult.
And leaving will be the same problem as getting there—it will
take at least an hour for the crowd to disperse."

I hung up in a wave of disappointment. I told myself to stop
this stupid self-pity. How could I be angry? It was Nelson
Mandela, after all. Security had to take priority over handicapped access. It wasn't the end of the world to miss a few
things, especially when I could see them on TV.

When I set about to contact the DisAbled Women's Network (DAWN) that summer, I was still pretending that it was
"research" for my book. But not too far below the surface,
I knew I was desperate to meet other women with disabilities, to see how they coped, what they thought, how their
lives with disability fit with their feminism.

DAWN Canada is a grassroots, self-help group formed to
make the disability movement more sensitive to women and
the women's movement more inclusive of disabled women.
I'd first heard of them when they approached Studio D to
make our screenings more accessible. We graciously acknowledged their criticism, and responded when it was
convenient, choosing the occasional wheelchair-accessible
venue, and enjoying the aesthetics of American Sign Lan-

guage at our movies; a low-cost way for us non-disabled feminists to feel righteous. But sometimes their demands seemed excessive, even strident, in view of all the other urgent items on our feminist agenda, the ones which seemed to affect *most* of us, rather than just a handful of unfortunate women.

Now I was embarrassed to remember my attitude. Only a year and a half earlier, fresh out of hospital and using a wheelchair myself, I had chosen a theater with inaccessible toilets to premiere *Mile Zero*. The ensuing months of curbs and stairs had shifted my priorities without my even noticing.

There was no listing for DAWN in the Montreal directory. I tried to reach something listed as the Handicapped Information and Referral Service and eventually talked to a person who informed me that the service no longer existed due to lack of funds. It was a harsh introduction to the economics of disability. I finally found the number of DAWN's national office—which turned out to be the kitchen table of the current Chair. She gave me a Montreal contact number and a meeting was set up at the local YWCA.

I almost didn't go. I felt tentative, apologetic about my status as a formerly "able-bodied" woman. I felt illegitimate because I was not as severely disabled as some other people. I felt guilty about the privileges of class, career, and family that made my experience so much easier than that of many others. I was a newcomer to the disability movement, while many women had already been working hard on my behalf; I had not paid my dues. (Doesn't this litany sound just like a woman?)

But my sister Razelle, who was visiting at the time, insisted I go. It would be good for me, she wisely said. She would go with me. So, hiding behind my sister and my tape recorder, I went to my first meeting of disabled feminists.

Like the Israeli Women's Network gathering, it was a small group of women, but this time I wasn't the only person who came in a wheelchair. We were a motley—some might say wretched—bunch who seemed to have little in common except our diverse disabilities, which turned out to be quite enough. I was not Other because here everyone was Other.

It was like the early days of consciousness-raising in the Women's Movement: those "clicks" of recognition, seeing yet again that the personal is political because disability, like gender, race, age, and sexuality is a social as well as biological construct. We shared painful and funny experiences, swapping practical tips about how to deal with local bureaucracies and which brand of tampons were least uncomfortable for constant sitting.

I learned that the three years it had taken me to begin to search out other people with disabilities was quite typical. Perhaps it's the time required to go through the various stages of loss. It may also be the time it takes to explore and ultimately exhaust the medical routes to rehabilitation. When I ventured hesitantly that perhaps I wasn't disabled enough, they all broke out laughing. "Almost everyone thinks they're not the real thing, because there's always someone else who's in even worse shape."

The biggest lesson, and most chastening, was to make

this connection with women who had not been part of my world before—women of different classes, women with less education, women with unusual physical "abnormalities" from whom I once would have averted my eyes in polite embarrassment. Most of the women were unemployed and poor. DAWN's research shows that 74 percent of women with disabilities are unemployed; 58 percent of women with disabilities live on less than $10,000 a year; and 23 percent of those women live on less than $5,000. Most of the women here were single and living with their parents.

One young woman with intellectual and emotional disabilities told us about having been abused by family members and caregivers. Women and children with disabilities are twice as vulnerable to violence as their non-disabled counterparts, yet very few rape crisis centers and shelters are accessible. Another woman told of her unsuccessful struggle to keep her children after she became physically disabled; their alcoholic father was considered a better parent.

I discovered that DAWN was not only a support group but part of a growing disability rights movement. People with disabilities were joining together to demand access and to claim their basic human rights.

The barriers that had kept me so firmly isolated from the other *bénéficiaires* at the Institut no longer seemed so insurmountable. What was the difference? Perhaps it was that we all identified as feminists. And maybe I no longer had to fight so hard against identifying myself as disabled.

Journal: June 28, 1990

It was with mixed feelings that I passed my driving test yesterday. I took the test without the manual controls, so my license
will be a regular one, not one that restricts me to an adapted
car. I feel as if I conned the OT into passing me without the re-
striction. I can't picture myself driving. But Michael is
concerned that we find some way to increase my autonomy before we leave for his sabbatical in September. We will be going
from city to city as he studies qualitative research techniques
and scouts out job possibilities, and I don't want to be
stranded when he is busy.

I can't believe I didn't get a scooter for three years. It
was Michael who pushed me to investigate those weird
three-wheeled things I had seen at the rehab center after
my first driving test. We had not seen one since, probably
because they're not paid for by Quebec provincial health
insurance.

I had bought the argument that a motorized vehicle
would be "giving up," something I would never do. Michael
persisted. He found a scooter distributor in one of the shopping malls. I resisted. He insisted. I tried one and it felt
unstable. I was scared of its powerful movement and unaccustomed speed. I felt like I was careening down the sidewalk
on a motorcycle, when in actuality its top pace was a Lucy-
trot. It felt so unprotected compared to an automobile, so
vulnerable. "But it's not meant for dodging through traffic,
only for sidewalks," the sales people argued.

Michael was sold; in fact, he was desperate. He saw its

potential when I could see only its finality. He dubbed it my "Freedom Machine." I called it "the Machine." I would later call her Gladys, after a suffragette's first bicycle, which she learned to ride at age fifty-three, but it took almost a year to achieve that level of intimacy, or even friendship.

My manual wheelchair had a sling-back and seat made of flexible nylon, which provided no support and no lever-age for wheeling myself. I sat low and slumped, a strained position for my back and neck. And I slumped even more when someone pushed me. I hated nagging about where I was placed: move me a little closer, a little further away, I'm blocking that entrance, I'M IN THE WAY.

The scooter on the other hand was *sportif*. My self-image changed. I sat straight and high. Most important, I determined exactly where I wanted to be and when. True, it was bulky and took more space, and I bumped into walls and sometimes even people, especially when going in re-verse. (Why did it take four years for us to figure out I could use a bicycle mirror?)

When I first tried to drive it, I was frightened of the smallest grade and of cars darting out of driveways, and made Michael walk beside me. It was months before I would cross a street alone; curb-cuts seemed steep and bumpy, and I worried that traffic couldn't see me because I was lower than cars. But my horizon was expanded far beyond what my limited strength for wheeling a manual chair had allowed. I could select my own clothing in department stores and roam the aisles of supermarkets, ferrying items from my basket to Michael's shopping cart. I could visit friends who lived within scooting range.

Best of all, I could just take a walk (a scoot?) with Lucy and enjoy being alone.

Journal: September 27, 1990
I was determined to use my new scooter as a convenience, but not as a substitute for rehab. We decided I should get a full re-assessment before we leave on sabbatical, so I called the Institut and discovered Michel Danakas was back from his sick leave and keen to work with me again.

After an hour of tests, Michel asked how much further I thought I would go. I responded that I've learned not to look towards an end point but to just notice the ongoing progress and accept each step forward as it comes. Once rhetoric, this is now truth, with momentary lapses and grief about loss.

I asked Michel to tell me how far *he* thought I would go. At first he tried to avoid my question. I persisted. I think he sensed that I was ready to hear what he thinks.

"What is it you really want to know?" he asked.

"Do you think I'll walk without canes?"

"No, at this point I'd have to say I can't see it."

It was so direct and bare—the first time I heard it. Or the first time I let myself hear it so clearly? I teared up, but I didn't feel devastated. I was sad but not surprised. I heard myself saying I could live with that, canes aren't so bad, I have a pretty good life.

Journal: October 4, 1990
I woke up today—the morning of our departure for Boston, first

stop on Michael's sabbatical—knowing that I won't ever walk unsupported. It doesn't feel heavy, though my voice choked when I tried to tell Michael. I have a big investment in positive thinking and imagining. But why do I still think of walking as the ultimate success? Walking is convenient, not essential. Now it seems appropriate to get on with my life. I don't want to make a career of rehabilitation. I won't stop trying; I think I can become more stable and comfortable. I have to figure out some weight-bearing exercises to combat the increased threat of osteoporosis that faces menopausal women who use wheelchairs. I'm looking forward to meeting more people with disabilities: learning how they live their lives, and finding out what other devices are available like my nerve-racking but liberating new scooter.

It took us all day to make the five-hour trip to Boston, with frequent stops for peeing, rest, and exercise. I had one bad moment in the car. All of a sudden my foot wouldn't move at all—oh no! that familiar feeling, stuck in paralysis. I looked before I panicked, and saw I was indeed stuck—with chewing gum on my sneaker.

Journal: October 10, 1990
Our first weekend in Boston. Naomi came from Toronto, and we decided to do the tourist thing, tooling around Boston Common. Michael and Naomi were on foot, I was on my new scooter. I was amazed to see so many wheelchairs and other vehicles—including what I've since learned are called "sip and puff" chairs which are controlled by breath, and special rigs for disabled children. "What an accessible city!" I sang happily.

Then we came upon a series of information tables—flyers, petitions, the familiar signs of a demonstration. The first table was an organization working to defeat a proposed bill which would make profound funding cutbacks for personal attendant care and sign language interpretation. The next table was for the Boston Self-Help Center, run by people with disabilities, who counsel each other and figure out what they need to live independently. How different from the demeaning charity stereotypes we're used to! Someone approached us with pins for sale: "Piss on Pity," "Nursing Homes Kill," "Label Cans, Not People" and "Disabled Dykes Do it with a Difference."

We had stumbled (wheeled?) into Boston's first annual Disability Pride Day! This was no casual coincidence of wheelchairs—this was a movement. Disability groups of all kinds were here, in coalition with trade unions, AIDS groups, and an assortment of progressive organizations. I was overcome, my belief in serendipity confirmed. Naomi grabbed Michael's camera and a notebook and was off to cover this event for her university newspaper.

A gutsy and nervous young woman with the thick drawl of cerebral palsy was emcee. Not only was her voice different, but there was a whole new language being spoken here. I felt like a privileged eavesdropper at first, but at the same time she was speaking for me and about me.

She cued us for a chant: "DISABLED AND . . . " The crowd responded: "PROUD!" My throat jammed on the word mid-chant. Is this honest? Who am I trying to fool? It's one thing to accept, but another to be proud. Proud of what? Of something I had nothing to do with? I'm proud of surviving and adapting maybe, but am I proud of being disabled? But it felt good to be shouting with hundreds of other bodies, looking happy in spite of—because of?—their deformities.

Or should I say "differences?" *Our* differences.

➤ Interlude: The Dancer Inside ➤

Journal: Vancouver, April, 1992

Independence '92, an historic moment in the disability community and, for me, my first professional work since *Mile Zero*, four years ago. I had hoped the media would be flooded with news of this, the first international conference on disability, with over 2,000 delegates from almost 100 countries. Instead, I found myself the only member of the Canadian national media present. I had convinced CBC radio to send me as a participant/documentarist. I felt very competent astride Gladys, my tape recorder in her basket, earphones on my head, and wires hanging off of me, but also pretty nervous. I'd never worked in radio before. I was unsure of the equipment, my capability, my stamina. The first night, exhausted from the trip, I lost my balance and fell in my hotel room, my worst fall in months. I lay on the floor crying into my tape recorder about what a mistake this all was. Why hadn't I asked Terre or Dorothy to co-direct? But in the morning I knew why.

I had never seen anything like it—nobody had, because nothing like it ever happened before. It was our world, for the next few days. We were a people, a nation, a tribe: with our own culture, history, heroes; our own languages; our own irreverent, rude humor, our own poets and artists. My eyes feasted on the images; so many sizes and shapes and kinds—gridlocks of wheelchairs, knocking into each other like bumper cars; wild arms waving for ASL, guide dogs leading chains of people, one arm on the shoulder in front of them like a train. I was wide-eyed in my ignorance as I was introduced to people whose disabilities were invisible or hidden—like epilepsy, learning disabilities, environmental sensitivities. We widened the circle to include people with chronic pain and illnesses like AIDS, and people who called themselves "psychiatric survivors"—contesting traditional definitions of mental illness. I discovered that our disability rights movement is international, its goals and priorities differing from culture to culture. I felt that we were making a revolution, creating a world in which disability is not a problem but part of the solution.

I was overwhelmed by the resourcefulness and creativity of the people I met. Here were rolling models galore. It was a supermarket of conveyances—from the fanciest motorized chairs to a legless Russian navigating a wheeled board with his hands on the floor at breakneck speed. So many variations on the theme of disability, people so different from me and people so like me. Where was my camera!

Why was this the first time I had seen someone in a wheelchair nursing a baby? Why weren't there pictures of us everywhere? Our visual absence breeds fear, breeds shame.

For many years I made films in which people who were invisible or misrepresented in our culture could see themselves. *Not a Love Story* charted the ways sexist pornography teaches us to hate our women's bodies. Now I was recognizing the ways in which society's ignorance and distorted images of disability have taught us people with disabilities to hate our bodies. This crowd of exuberant freaks taught me something different: something like pride.

The climax of the conference for me was a performance by three Brazilian dancers: a young girl, about ten, in a silver wheelchair; a thin, muscular woman in a wheelchair with day-glo yellow wheels; and a non-disabled woman with a mane of curly black hair. One dancer climbed under and over the chairs while another pivoted around her, pulling herself into the air, borrowing balance from the third and then tipping the silver chair to spill them all to the ground where they mingled arms, legs, torsos, not fighting gravity but dancing with it. There was nothing odd-looking about it. One woman used her legs, the other two couldn't—what could be more natural? They danced, powerfully, sensuously. We all have a primal instinct and desire to communicate, even when many of our abilities are taken away from us. Maybe when the clutter of life is gone, we're free to discover its essence.

Afterwards I interviewed the Brazilian women and then I shyly asked if I could dance with them myself. I put my canes aside. I was leaning on Rosangela, the non-disabled dancer, with every part of my body. She was giving me cues, whispering in my ear in her sultry voice: "Relax your head, lend me your arms, lean on me, trust my body, my legs will be your legs."

I let go and trusted. We moved fast and wild. I heard myself screaming with joy. I had no idea what it looked like nor did I care. The dancer inside me was out.

➳ Epilogue: On a Roll ➳

Here I am, back in my "outdoor office," the ground around me littered with cherry blossoms. So much has changed since I began writing this book. Lucy no longer lies patiently by my paisley scooter, dreaming dog dreams. She died of old age, and I have since raised a new puppy, Louie, to be my companion dog. The original Gladys is retired to the country.

Slow Dance ends three years after my stroke, when I accepted that I would be permanently disabled. After a few more housebound years in Montreal, I was relieved when Michael found a challenging position as Head of Family Practice at the B.C. Women's and B.C. Children's Hospitals, and we were able to move to the disability-friendly city of Vancouver.

Happily, Seth joined us on the coast and is now coordinating a research center on social policy alternatives. Naomi is a newspaper columnist in Toronto and is writing a book about anti-corporate activism. Both our children are beginning families of their own. Michael's parents, Annie and Philip, traded rural New Jersey for B.C.'s fabled Sunshine Coast, a short ferry ride away from us.

As for me, getting around my Vancouver neighborhood is as easy as I could imagine! I scoot along the scenic bicycle paths, knowing I'll find ramps into most buildings and curb-cuts on most streets. I still don't drive a car, but some city buses are lift-equipped. We also have a customized transportation system known as Handidart, run by a board of people with disabilities, and a subsidized fleet of ramped taxicabs for even greater spontaneity.

This easy access means that I have a life. Besides seeing

family, friends, shul-mates, colleagues, and neighbors, I have a community of other people with disabilities: strangers in wheelchairs to beep to, close friends with whom to share my fears and triumphs, organizations like the B.C. Coalition of People with Disabilities and DAWN Canada with whom to think and advocate for our issues. The heady feelings of Independence '92 have given way to a more realistic sense of the work needed to build a strong human rights movement; this too is a long haul.

The stroke forced me to transform my life, to abandon the clock and calendar, and to heed my body's ever-changing requirements. I've learned to be more patient, as have those around me. I ration my limited energy and choose carefully who I see and what I do. Every day I swim, exercise, and nap. Every week I get body work—massage, chiropractic, acupuncture—to maximize fluidity and minimize pain. Once prescriptive, these rituals are now essential parts of my new life, a life that feels balanced and healthy.

I no longer consider myself in "rehabilitation," yet I am still progressing, almost eleven years after my stroke. The changes are subtle; perhaps only I can see them. Fortunately, I can afford to continually sample new approaches and teachers, to stimulate my mind and nervous system. The result is that I can stand comfortably—even dance—for longer stretches than before.

I also have rare moments of anger at my loss, and occasional tears. It seems unfair that, in light of my stroke, I was not exempted from aging! I went through menopause and have acquired osteoporosis and osteoarthritis in my lower back, both conditions probably caused by my enforced sitting.

People often ask whether I think about making films again. One of the great gifts of the stroke was the discovery that I can live well without the role or title of filmmaker. I'm happy to be known as Bonnie Sherr Klein, unlabelled and institution-free. I still have the desire to share what I am learning, maybe more than ever. Making documentaries for the CBC turned out to be a perfect adaptation to my new limitations. And writing this book has been even more stimulating and pleasureful.

Since the Canadian release of *Slow Dance,* both Michael and I have received many requests to consult and speak, in Canada and elsewhere. We share our stories with other stroke survivors and their families, disability groups, various health professionals, and the general community. When people tell us about their own experiences with severe and chronic illness, rehabilitation and disability, some common themes emerge.

When a person is very sick, they need a vigilant advocate—a family doctor and/or close family member or friend—to choreograph their path through the system: to interpret, question, and challenge. We've learned that whenever possible, a sick person should not be left alone in the hospital, but should receive constant support and care. *

Survivors and people with disabilities have discovered that we are the experts about our own bodies, and we must take charge of our lives. This means figuring out and asking for what we need, becoming actively involved in our own care and rehabilitation, seeking out peers and allies, joining with disability rights activists—and making a stink when necessary!

We need health professionals to listen well, to encourage

our hope, and to join us as allies. We like to remind health professionals, who seem more and more demoralized in whatever country we've found them, of the idealistic reasons why they entered their field in the first place.

Together we need to heal our health-care and rehabilitation systems, to promote a vision motivated not by the bottom line, but by a collective commitment to the best care for all.

∾

Before my stroke, I had a mistaken notion that feminism meant "independence;" the unspoken corollary was that dependence on others is shameful. What I've learned finally is that in asking for help I offer other people an opportunity for intimacy and collaboration. Whether I'm asking for me personally or for disabled people collectively, I give them the opportunity to be their most human. In Judaism, we call this gift a mitzvah.

Who would have dreamed that my stroke would have brought me to this moment, this place, this park bench? Gladys II is parked next to me, still factory-bright. Michael suggests we paint her with spits of flame like a motorcycle. But Louie is restless now; he wants to roll in the grass and play catch in the nearby park. And so do I.

∾ Vancouver, Spring 1998

* Klein, Michael C., *"Too Close for Comfort? A family physician questions whether medical professionals should be excluded from their loved ones' care."* Canadian Medical Association Journal 1997; 156: 53-55.

❊ Acknowledgments ❊

I am deeply grateful to the many friends and relatives who played a role in my survival and recovery—only some of whom are mentioned in this book. You will never be forgotten.

~

Muriel Duckworth and Judy Steed first suggested I write a book. Many individuals encouraged and supported the idea, especially Leah Appet, Jeff Borkan, Leon Bibb, June Callwood, Sandra Campbell, Josh Freed, Ruth Hundert, Jackie Kaiser at Penguin Books, Gabor Kalman, Barbara Kay, Sheila Kitzinger, Abby Lippman, Barbara Pulling at Douglas & McIntyre, Shirley Turcotte, Patrick Watson, Anne Wheeler, and Merrily Weisbord.

The Canada Council Explorations Program, now regrettably defunct, funded the transcription of my journals and tapes. The transcribers were Nora Allyne, Lauren Banerd, Pat Billing, Gigi Grein, Kathleen Kelly, Eileen Lavery, and Irit Shimrat.

Susan Furze, an invaluable personal assistant during that crucial first year in Vancouver, organized my office and computer system.

Several brave souls tried to teach me computer skills: Andy Orkin, Bill Lake, and especially Lani Levine, who insists that I am "not stupid, just slow," and promises to teach me how to transfer files without taxicabs.

My daughter Naomi Klein accompanied me back to

the Jewish General Hospital and Institut de Réadaptation de Montréal to interview staff, read and indexed the transcripts of my journals, and helped me to see the book not as a dwelling on the painful past but a bridge to my future.

My agent, Denise Bukowski, was indefatigable. Janet Turnbull Irving offered generous advice.

Knopf publisher Louise Dennys, who believed in the book before I'd written a word, supported me with patience and edited with brilliance and tact; Bernice Eisenstein thinned the ponderous first draft; and Diane Martin clarified the manuscript with loving care.

People in the disability rights and writing community became my mentors and friends, and informed my disability consciousness: Marsha Saxton, who helped me understand both disability oppression and liberation; Nancy Mairs, who writes so personally and truthfully about all the bad stuff as well as the blessings of being disabled; Jean Stewart, who offered valuable guidelines after reading a very early stage of this manuscript; Judy Heumann, a leader in the international disability rights movement, now U.S. Assistant Secretary of Education; Ed Roberts, a gutsy pioneer in the independent living movement, and Irving Kenneth Zola, an original thinker and leader in the disability studies and self-help movements, both deceased; Susan Harkins, my "stroke sister," who is now surviving an even crueller stroke; Joan Meister, who urged us to move to Vancouver, and Carol Herbert, who helped make it happen; and Maxine Tynes, poet, who confirmed the need to tell our stories at a Women In View workshop, "The Writer as Social Activist."

For sharing their firsthand knowledge of disability, I thank: Sally Aitken, Gerald Batista, Margaret Birrell, Mary Lou Breslin, Diane Dolan, Ellen Frank, Susan Griffin, Jan Hamilton, Ronnie Wenker Konner, Mark Limont, Diane Lipton Armstrong, Bill Livant, Margot Massie, Shirley Masuda, Pauline Rankin, Connie Rockwood, Susan Wendell, Ellen Wiebe, Mary Williams, and the many people who participated in Marsha Saxton's co-counselling workshops for people with disabilities and allies.

For reading the manuscript at various stages: Ruth Nemzoff Berman, Sherry Bie, Dr. Betty Callum, Diane Carrière, Ellen Frank, Razelle Frankl, Jan Hamilton, Dorothy Todd Hénaut, Anne Henderson, Dr. Carol Herbert, Signe Johansson, Sidonie Kerr, Mark Limont, Della McCreary, Joan Meister, Gaby Minnes, Terre Nash, Eileen O'Brien, Gerry Rogers, Marsha Saxton, Kathleen Shannon, Dr. Ellen Wiebe, Norma Zack, Lillian Zimmerman, and all my family.

For the Hasidic story, Reb Hillel Goelman and Leonard Angel.

Thanks to the Canadian Association of Occupational Therapists for inviting me to be keynote speaker at their annual conference; and to Tim Readman, Sandra Bressler, and especially Dr. Helene Polatajko for our Crawford Lectureship dialogue about synergistic therapist-client relationships.

CBC radio colleagues: Nancy Watson, Joe Moulins, Peter Leo, Shelley Pomerantz, David Gutnick, Peter Gzowski,

Stuart McLean, and especially Alex Frame, who had the vision and provided the support; hurrah for public broadcasting!

Robin Morgan at Ms. magazine, for commissioning my first article, "We Are Who You Are: Feminism and Disability;" Judy Razminsky for editing it; and Shirley Masuda for the title.

My co-counsellors Claire Kujundzik, Bill Horne, and especially Elizabeth Shefrin, with whom I retrieved some important memories.

My son Seth Klein and his "farm" friends.

For holding body and soul together: massage therapists Coleen Quinn, Vicki Hall, Mary Boulding, Kendall Dixon; cranial therapist Patricia Pucher; Alexander teachers Lyn Charlsen, Gabriella Minnes Brandes; chiropractors Jean Chevrefils and Aaron Hoy; naturopath Eric Posen; and family physician Joy Russell.

People who loaned us their homes as writing retreats and nurtured us: Lanie Melamed, Rob Melamed, Rhema Cossover, Isadora's Restaurant, Cora Domingo, and especially Annie and Philip Klein.

Sun-Life for excellent service with my disability insurance.

Special thanks to Nenelle and Brad Bunnin for the connection to PageMill Press, to Jennifer Shepherd for the contract, to Nancy Pollak for this edit, and to Roy M. Carlisle and the team at Circulus Publishing Group, Inc., home of PageMill Press and Wildcat Canyon Press.

Persimmon would like to thank Della McCreary for listening to each revision of every chapter, hot off the computer. Her complex perspectives on disability combined with her love of words made for invaluable feedback.

Persimmon would also like to thank Bonnie Sherr Klein for more than is possible to list here, but most especially for the irrepressible exuberance she brought to even the most picky parts of this process.

❧ Recommended Reading ❧

These are books on illness or disability—both fiction and non-fiction, personal and general—that I found useful, illuminating or inspiring.

Allende, Isabel. Margaret S. Peder trans. *Paula.* (New York: HarperCollins, 1995).

Asch, Adrienne and Michelle Fine. *Women with Disabilities: Essays in Psychology, Politics, and Policy.* (Philadelphia: Temple University Press, 1988).

Blackbridge, Persimmon. *Sunnybrook: A True Story with Lies.* (Vancouver: Press Gang Publishers, 1996).

Blackbridge, Persimmon, and Sheila Gilhooly. *Still Sane.* (Vancouver: Press Gang Publishers, 1985).

Borysenko, Joan. *Minding the Body, Mending the Mind.* (New York: Bantam Books, 1988).

Brown, Susan E., Debra Connors, and Nancy Stern, eds. *With the Power of Each Breath: A Disabled Woman's Anthology.* (Pittsburgh: Cleis Press, 1985).

Cousins, Norman. *Anatomy of an Illness as Perceived by the Patient: Reflections on Healing and Regeneration.* (New York: W.W. Norton & Co, Inc., 1979).

Finger, Anne. *Past Due: A Story of Disability, Pregnancy, and Birth.* (Seattle: Seal Press, 1990).

Frank, Arthur W. *The Wounded Storyteller: Body, Illness, and Ethics.* (Chicago: University of Chicago Press, 1995).

Frankl, Viktor. *Man's Search for Meaning.* (New York: Pocket Books, 1985).

Goffman, Erving. *Stigma: Notes on the Management of Spoiled Identity.* (New York: Simon & Schuster, 1963).

Heilbrun, Carolyn G. *Writing a Woman's Life*. (New York: W.W. Norton & Co., Inc., 1988).

Heymann, Jody, M.D. *Equal Partners: A Physician's Call For a New Spirit of Medicine*. (New York: Little Brown & Co., 1995).

Hillyer, Barbara. *Feminism & Disability*. (Norman, Oklahoma: University of Oklahoma Press, 1993).

Hockenberry, John. *Moving Violations: War Zones, Wheelchairs and Declarations of Independence*. (New York: Hyperion, 1995).

Hull, John M. *Touching the Rock: An Experience of Blindness*. (New York: Pantheon Books, 1990).

Kleinman, Arthur. *The Illness Narratives*. (New York: Basic Books, 1988).

Lear, Martha Weinman. *Heartsounds: The Story of a Love and Loss*. (New York: Simon & Schuster, 1980).

Levine, Stephen. *Healing into Life and Death*. (New York: Anchor Press, Doubleday, 1987).

Lorde, Audre. *A Burst of Light*. (Ithaca, New York: Firebrand Books, 1988).

Mairs, Nancy. *Carnal Acts*. (New York: HarperCollins, 1990).

—*Plaintext: Deciphering a Woman's Life*. (Tucson: University of Arizona Press, 1986).

—*Remembering the Bone House: An Erotics of Place and Space*. (New York: Harper & Row, 1988).

—*Voice Lessons: On Becoming a (Woman) Writer*. (Boston: Beacon Press, 1994).

—*Waist-High in the World: A Life among the Nondisabled*. (Boston: Beacon Press, 1997).

Morris, Jenny. *Pride against Prejudice: Transforming Attitudes toward Disability*. (Philadelphia: New Society Pubs., 1993).

Morris, Jenny, ed. *Able Lives: Women's Experience of Paralysis*. (London: The Women's Press, 1989).

Murphy, Robert F. *The Body Silent.* (New York: Henry Holt & Co., 1987).

Panzarino, Connie. *The Me in the Mirror.* (Seattle: Seal Press, 1994).

Sacks, Oliver. *The Man Who Mistook His Wife for a Hat.* (New York: HarperCollins, 1987).

—*A Leg to Stand On.* (New York: HarperCollins, 1994).

—*An Anthropologist on Mars: Seven Paradoxical Tales.* (Toronto: Alfred A. Knopf Canada, 1995).

Saxton, Marsha and Florence Howe, eds. *With Wings: An Anthology of Literature by and about Women with Disabilities.* (New York: Feminist Press at the City University, 1988).

Shapiro, Joseph P. *No Pity: People with Disabilities Forging a New Civil Rights Movement.* (New York: Times Books, 1993).

Shaw, Barrett, ed. *The Ragged Edge: The Disability Experience from the Pages of the First Fifteen Years of The Disability Rag.* (Advocado Press, 1994. (P.O. Box 145, Louisville, KY 40201-0145)).

Sontag, Susan. *Illness as Metaphor.* (New York: St. Martin's Press, 1989).

Stewart, Jean. *The Body's Memory.* (New York: St. Martin's Press, 1989).

Wendell, Susan. *The Rejected Body: Feminist Philosophical Reflections on Disability.* (New York: Routledge, 1996).

Zola, Irving Kenneth. *Missing Pieces: A Chronicle of Living with a Disability.* (Philadelphia: Temple University Press, 1982).

Zola, Irving Kenneth, ed., *Ordinary Lives: A Collection of Voices of Disability and Disease.* (Cambridge/Watertown, Mass.: Apple-wood Books, 1982).

❋ Biographies ❋

Bonnie Sherr Klein is one of Canada's best-known documentary filmmakers, infamous internationally for *Not a Love Story: A Film about Pornography*. She was the subject of her own award-winning CBC radio series, *Bonnie & Gladys,* in which she explored being a person with a disability. She gets around with two canes or on Gladys (her motorized scooter). As passionate an activist as ever, she now counsels and speaks about health care, rehabilitation and disability rights. She lives in Vancouver and on the Sunshine Coast with her husband, Michael.

Persimmon Blackbridge, with whom Bonnie Klein collaborated in the writing of *Slow Dance,* is a visual artist and writer. Her most recent novel is *Prozac Highway* (Press Gang, 1997).

PageMill Press publishes books primarily in the field of psychology, with an eye to personal growth. Our authors explore the intellectual, psychological, and spiritual dimensions of our daily lives—the connection between mind and body, the power of myth and dreams in everyday circumstances, the role of the unconscious in human interactions, the wisdom and insight the body has to offer our total health, and the integration of a fuller experience of the body in life's activities.

For a catalog of our publications or editorial submissions, please write:

PAGEMILL PRESS
2716 Ninth Street
Berkeley, CA 94710
Phone: (510) 848-3600
Fax: (510) 848-1326
E-mail: Circulus@aol.com